Good Carb, Bad Carb
For a Healthy Lifestyle

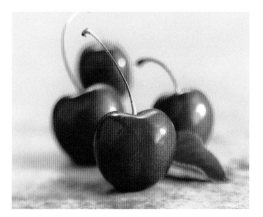

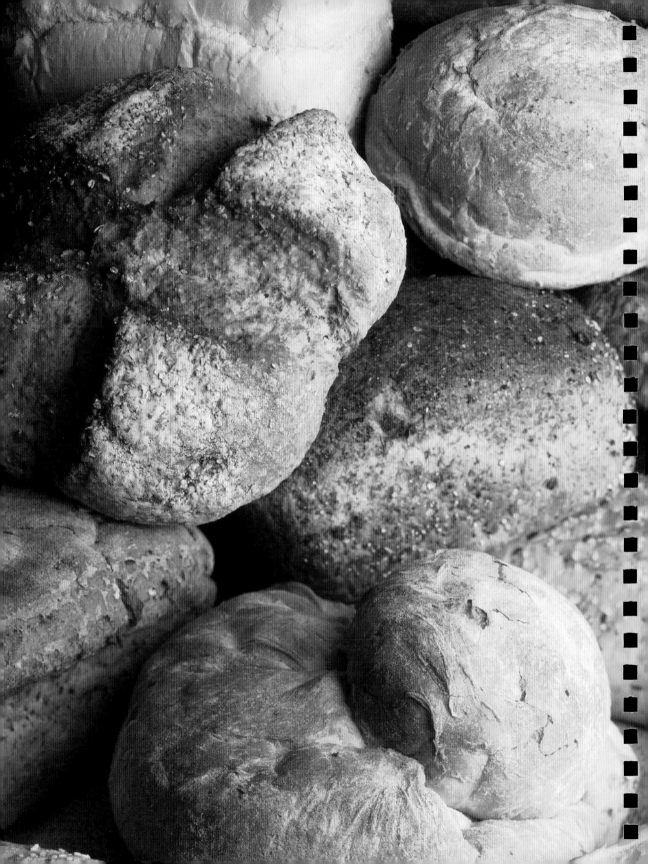

Good Carb, Bad Carb

For a Healthy Lifestyle

IMPROVE YOUR DIET

NUTRITIONAL FACTS

STEP-BY-STEP RECIPES

Wynnie Chan

Main Street
A division of Sterling Publishing Co., Inc.
New York

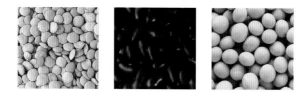

Library of Congress Cataloging-in-Publication Data Available

10 9 8 7 6 5 4 3 2 1

Published by Main Street, a division of Sterling Publishing Co., Inc.
387 Park Avenue South, New York, NY 10016
© 2005 by PRC Publishing

An imprint of **Chrysalis** Books Group plc

Distributed in Canada by Sterling Publishing
c/o Canadian Manda Group, 165 Dufferin Street
Toronto, Ontario, Canada M6K 3H6

Printed in China

ISBN 1 4027 1963 9

Every effort has been made to trace the ownership of all copyrighted
material and to secure permission from copyright holders. In the
eventof any question arising as to the use of any material,
we will be pleased to make necessary corrections in future printings.

This book is not intended to replace expert medical advice. The author and
the publisher urge you to verify the appropriateness of any diet with your
qualified health care professional, especially if you have any existing
medical conditions, are taking any medications, are pregnant, or nursing.
The author and the publisher disclaim any liability or loss, personal or
otherwise, resulting from the procedures and information in this book.

All measurements are approximate and in the case of processed foods,
can vary between brands.

Contents

Carbs: The simple facts

Carbs

the simple facts

If you look through any newspaper or magazine today, you will undoubtedly find a myriad of low-carb diet plans, which promise miraculous weight loss and countless health benefits. In many of these diets, the so-called "bad" carbs are blamed for a multitude of sins. But is it right to assume that such a generalizing statement is true?

what are carbohydrates?

We all need energy to perform vital functions, whether we are walking, running, eating, sleeping, thinking, or just breathing. Food provides us with the energy we require; but while some would say we eat to live, others would say we live to eat.

Carbohydrates are one of the three major groups of nutrients that provide us with that energy, protein and fat are the other two (alcohol also provides energy but it isn't classed as an essential nutrient!). Carbohydrates are, in fact, the primary source of energy (or fuel) for the cells and organs in our body. The brain, nervous system, muscles, and red blood cells all rely on a constant supply of carbohydrates in the form of glucose (sugar) to remain active. Every gram of carbohydrate provides us with four calories of energy (protein also yields four calories per gram and alcohol seven calories, while fat is a much more concentrated energy source, providing nine calories per gram).

Carbs can also be stored in the body as glycogen, in the muscles and liver. This reserve of carbs can be utilized by the body to maintain a steady supply of glucose at times when our diet does not supply enough. For example, when we are asleep or during times when we are sick and cannot eat. The store of glycogen in the liver is used up quickly and on average it lasts for about 18 hours, after which point our body has to create its own carbs from dietary protein.

where do carbohydrates come from?

We rely on the humble plant to provide us with the majority of carbohydrates in our food as the only animal products that contain carbs are milk and dairy products.

Carbs are made up of three elements: carbon, hydrogen, and oxygen, which are all bound together with energy-containing bonds. Through a process called photosynthesis,

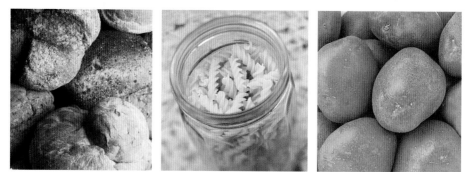

plants take carbon dioxide (from the air), water, and energy (from the sun) and use them as the basic ingredients to form carbohydrates.

Foods can contain two different types of carbohydrates. To make these, the three elements that form carbohydrates (carbon, hydrogen, and oxygen) are arranged in different orders. Simple carbohydrates, as the term suggests, have a very simple chemical structure and can usually be broken down (or digested) easily.

Did You Know?

Carbo means carbon and *hydrate* means from water.

Complex carbohydrates, obviously, have a more complicated chemical structure and therefore it takes our body a lot longer to digest them.

simple carbohydrates in food

Simple carbohydrates include sugars such as glucose, fructose (fruit sugar), and galactose. These are known as monosaccharides (*mono* = one or single and *saccharide* = sugar). Glucose, also referred to as blood sugar, is the main monosaccharide found in the body that provides us with fuel. Single sugars, such as glucose, can be joined together to make double sugars or disaccharides (*di* = two, *saccaharide* = sugar). These sugars include:

- *Sucrose.* A combination of glucose and fructose. This is the common table sugar found in sugar cane, sugar beets, honey, and maple syrup.
- *Lactose.* This is glucose and galactose combined. It is known commonly as milk sugar and is found in milk and dairy products.
- *Maltose.* This is made up of two glucose units joined together and is used in making alcohol.

When you eat a foods that contain single sugars, they are absorbed rapidly into your bloodstream. When you eat a food that contains dissacharides, your body has to break them down to single sugars first before they can be absorbed into your bloodstream. Once dissacharides are broken down into single sugars, most are transformed into glucose in the liver. The table on the right is a list of simple sugars that are used both as ingredients in foods and are also available to buy in most grocery stores.

Label Lingo?

Food products that list simple sugars among the first few ingredients contain substantial amounts per serving. If you are watching your weight or trying to cut down on sugars, check the labels carefully before you buy.

Simple or added sugars
white or regular sugar
brown sugar
molasses
confectioner's sugar (finely powdered sucrose)
corn syrup or corn sweetener
honey
maple syrup
fruit juice concentrate
high-fructose corn syrup
granulated sugar
invert sugar
glucose (dextrose)
fructose
lactose
maltose
fruit sugar
palm sugar
date sugar
rock sugar
caramel
dextrose
polydextrose
sorbitol
levulose

complex carbohydrates in food

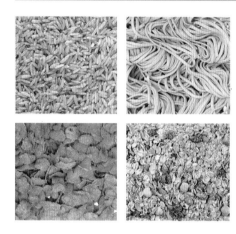

Complex carbs are sometimes referred to as polysaccharides (*poly* = many and *saccharide* = sugar). These carbs are made up of many simple sugars joined together with energy-containing bonds. Starch is one example of a complex carb found in foods; humans store glucose as glycogen, while plants store glucose as starch. Some complex carbs are indigestible and are known as fiber. Examples of starchy foods include:

- breads
- cereals
- crackers
- rice
- pasta
- noodles
- oatmeal
- bulghur
- quinoa
- millet

As you may have guessed, unlike simple carbs, complex carbs require our body to expend a lot more energy to digest them. Digestion of a complex carb, like starch, starts as soon as you place it in your mouth and begin chewing. An

enzyme in your saliva, called amylase, initially attacks the starch by breaking down some of the long chains of sugars into smaller chains.

Next, the food (now consisting of smaller chains of sugars, plus fiber and some long chains of sugars) is pushed down into the stomach and mixed with acids and digestive juices before traveling to the small intestine. Here another enzyme breaks down the remaining starch into smaller chains of sugars and double sugars. Before these sugars can be absorbed into the bloodstream they have to undergo one last split into single sugars. This happens in the lining of the small intestine.

These remaining single sugars are then carried to the liver by the blood, where they are converted into glucose if needed, or into fats and taken to the body's cells to be used for fuel or stored. The liver and muscles also store some glucose as glycogen and then change it back to glucose when needed. Fiber passes unchanged (undigested) and so at this stage it may appear to be an unnecessary nutrient but, as discussed in the next chapter, it can be seen as a detoxifying agent.

Sugar alcohols, such as sorbitol, are the most widely used sweeteners found in "diabetic" food. These have similar functions to most sugars. As is the case with normal sugars, they raise blood sugar levels and contain calories. Although sorbitol contains slightly less calories than glucose, be careful as eating large quantities will result in frequent trips to the restroom (the reason why sorbitol has fewer calories is because it isn't completely digested, hence their laxative effect). Artificial or intense sweeteners, such as saccharin and aspartame, are not classified as carbohydrates and have no effect on blood glucose levels.

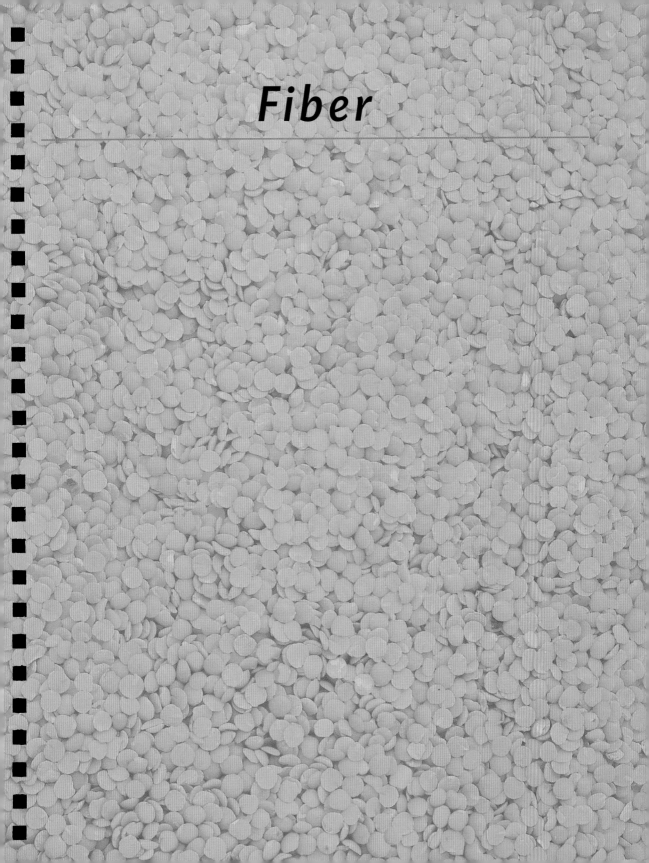

Fiber

Fiber

the cleansing nutrient

Fiber is a complex carbohydrate made up of long chains of sugars held together by bonds that the enzymes in our body cannot break down. Most of the fiber contained in food passes straight through our digestive tract without providing us with any energy. It does help to move things along in the gut though, so it is suitable to think of it as a detox ingredient.

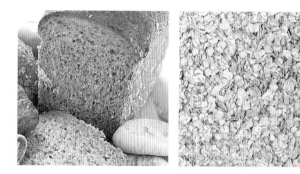

There are two types of fiber contained in the food that we eat:

- *Insoluble fiber*. This comes primarily from wholegrains and cereals, wheat and corn bran, green beans, potatoes, and the skins of fruits and vegetables. It does not dissolve in water.
- *Soluble fiber.* This is obtained from fruits, vegetables, oats, oat bran, barley, brown rice, beans, legumes, pulses, and pectin. This type of fiber does dissolve in water.

reasons to like fiber

It curbs your cravings for snacks
Fibers have the ability to absorb water like a sponge and swell up in your gut. It therefore fills you up for longer, so you are less likely to snack between meals.

It helps you to control your weight
Because fiber fills you up and you are less likely to want to snack on sugary and fatty foods, which are calorie-dense, you will naturally reduce your calorie intake. Fiber itself provides us with very little calories. Research has shown that the majority of people who follow high-fiber, low-fat diets generally weigh less than those who do not.

It keeps your gut healthy
Fiber has the ability to absorb water (much like a sponge) and it therefore helps you to keep the contents of your gut moist. This factor means that the body can eliminate stools more easily and this in itself can prevent or ease health problems such as hemorrhoids, diverticulosis (see next entry), and constipation.

It stimulates the muscles of the gut so that they retain their tone
This may help to prevent diverticulosis, a condition where areas of the gut wall balloon out as a the result of weakening of the intestinal muscles.

It reduces the risk of heart disease by lowering blood cholesterol
The bacteria that live in our gut can break down some types of soluble fiber producing small fat-like compounds. These are thought to stop or reduce the liver's production of cholesterol. Research has proven that soluble fiber from oatmeal, called beta-glucan, helps to lower blood cholesterol. A health study (conducted in the U.S.) investigated the diets of a large group of women. They found that compared to those who had a low intake of wholegrains (less than one serving a day), women who ate, on average, $2^1/2$ servings of wholegrains everyday showed a 30 percent decrease in the risk of developing coronary heart disease.

It may decrease the risk of developing cancer

Insoluble fibers have the ability to bind or dilute cancer-causing compounds. The more fiber you eat, the quicker their transit (exit) time through the colon. A study published in 2002 concluded that people on a high-fiber diet (approx. 32.5g a day) reduced the chance of developing cancer of the colon by 40 percent compared to those with a low intake (approx. 12g). It also advised that eating fruit and vegetables (18 oz. or more a day) reduces the risk of developing cancer in the upper gastrointestinal tract by 50 percent.

Fiber can help diabetics to control their blood sugar levels

Research shows that soluble fiber has the ability to slow down the digestion of carbohydrates and absorbtion of glucose thus avoiding major blood sugar swings.

Remember: fruit and vegetable juices contain very little fiber so don't drink all of your fruit and vegetable portions in the form of juice as you will miss out on the benefits of the fiber fruits contain. You should limit your intake to one 6 oz. serving per day.

label lingo—what does it all mean?

Nutritional labels can often be confusing. Listed below is a quick guide to some of the terms and their translations:

Enriched U.S. law requires that specific levels of thiamin, riboflavin, niacin, folate, and iron be added to refined grains and grain products.

Refined flour This means that the outer parts of wheat (bran, husk, and germ) have been removed during milling to make regular white flour.

Wheat flour Any flour made from wheat, including regular white flour, can be called wheat flour.

Husk The outer (inedible) part of a grain.

Bran This is the fibrous coating around a grain.

Endosperm The starchy (edible) part of a grain.

Wholegrain Not refined. Grain (not the husk) is milled in its entirety.

Whole-wheat Wholegrain flour made from whole-wheat kernels.

Fortified Some grain foods are fortified with folate or folic acid, sometimes called folacin, a B group vitamin that prevents birth defects.

On the right are examples of a refined and an unrefined breakfast cereal to illustrate the differences in nutritional contents.

How Much Fiber Do You Need?

Health professionals recommend around 20–35g of fiber a day. Most Americans eat around 11g, which is a lot less than this. Generally, men should eat 30–38g a day, while women should aim for a daily intake of 21–25g. Children of course need less fiber than this. Most experts recommend a fiber intake of "age + 5." For example, if your child is six, then they require 6+5 = 11 grams a day.

Did You Know?

Nutrition panels on labels sometimes detail the amount of insoluble and soluble fiber. Usually only the total amount contained per serving is listed. As a rule, food containing 2.5g of fiber per serving is a "good" source of fiber.

	100g unrefined cereal	100g refined cereal
Energy	1400kj/ 330cal	1643kj/ 388cal
Protein	10g	6g
Carbohydrate	67g	83g
of which sugars	21g	34g
of which starch	46g	49g
Fat	2.0g	3.5g
of which saturates	0.3g	0.7g
Fiber	15g	2.5g
Sodium	0.75g	0.6g

13

how to add more fiber into your diet

- If you are used to eating sugar-coated refined cereals then it will take some time to adjust to eating high-fiber cereals. Start by replacing a quarter of your normal bowl of refined cereal with one that supplies around 2g of fiber per serving. That way you can gradually increase the amount of fiber-rich cereal you eat every day.
- Eliminate refined white rice from your diet and replace it with brown rice as a staple.

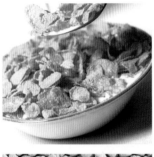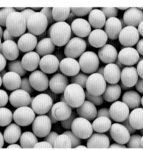
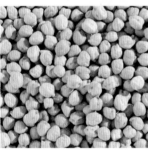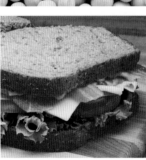

- If you love your sandwiches made with white bread, but want to reap the benefits from wholegrains, remove one slice of white and replace it with whole-wheat bread.
- Swap refined foods for unprocessed ones:
    a) Brown not white. Eat a slice of whole-wheat bread instead of white and gain

Label Lingo

Enriched white flour is sometimes listed as "wheat flour" on food labels. This is not the same as whole-wheat flour and so contains less fiber.

Did You Know?

The best thing since sliced *white* bread? That would be a bad comparison. Unlike wholegrain bread, unenriched white bread is devoid of iron, and the B vitamins, thiamin, riboflavin, and niacin.

an additional 4g of fiber. Or swap half a cup of boiled white rice for half a cup of boiled brown rice which will give you an extra 2g of fiber.

- b) Keep your skin on. Exchange half a cup of boiled mashed potatoes for a medium baked potato and you will gain an extra 3g of fiber.
- c) Bean not cream. Swap half a cup of sour cream dip for half a cup of bean dip and gain an additional 1.5 g of fiber.
- Try adding bran cereal to casseroles or baked vegetable dishes to give them a crunchy topping.
- Use the half and half concept. Bake your own bread and substitute half of all the white flour you use with wholegrain flour. (You might need to add a bit more yeast than usual.) If you are substituting wholegrain flour for white flour in baked goods, you will probably need to add a bit more baking powder. (1 tsp. extra for 3 cups of whole-wheat flour.)
- Experiment with different grains. Try brown rice, barley, whole-wheat pasta, bulgur, wild rice, and kasha—these will also add greater variety to your diet.
- When you are cooking spaghetti sauce, trying adding some vegetables as well. Not only will this increase the fiber content, but it will make the sauce go further.
- Try adding beans or lentils to soups or salads.
- Copy the Asian way of eating by finishing off your meals with fruit. Seasonal fruits make great economical and healthful choices.
- Flaxseeds are high in fiber and can be sprinkled over salads, soups, cereals, and yogurt to add fiber and extra flavor.

CASE STUDY: purified bran and bran supplements

Peter is a middle-aged man of average health. After reading a report in the newspaper about the benefits of increasing his fiber consumption he decided to buy some purified oat and wheat bran to mix in with his cereal in the morning. He reasoned that if some bran was good for him then more must be even better. He started to experiment with his recipes and added some purified wheat bran to his muffin mixture as well. Unfortunately, he ended up in the emergency room because his gut couldn't cope with the excessive amounts of purified fiber he was eating.

The warning:
Purified fibers should only ever be used in moderation. Your dietary fiber requirements are best met through eating an appropriate amount of fiber-rich whole foods and not through purified fibers and supplements.

Tip

Fiber isn't a miracle substance. It is only through its absence in refined foods that its importance becomes clear. So, go easy on the supplements.

CASE STUDY: very high fiber diets

Roberta is 80 years old, and suffers with hemorrhoids. She was advised by a friend that a high-fiber diet would help her condition, so she decided to eat bran cereals, bran muffins, rye bread, whole-wheat spaghetti, and anything she could find in her grocery store that was fiber-rich. Roberta didn't drink many cups of tea or glasses of water as she did not like having to go to the restroom too often. As a consequence of her new diet and low fluid intake she suffered from terrible gas and eventually ended up in the emergency room. It was revealed that she had been consuming an abnormally high amount of fiber—around 60g per day, which is more than double the recommended amount. Her intestine had become blocked with fiber balls, or phytobezoars, which had to be removed through surgery.

The warning:
Very high fiber diets can lead to problems for the elderly and people with diabetes because they can cause intestinal blockage, particularly if insufficient amounts of water are consumed.

Tip

You need to drink more fluids as you increase your fiber intake. This will then help the fiber pass more easily (and quickly) through the gut.

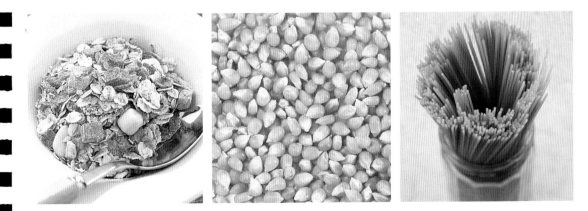

sources of fiber

Bread, cereals, rice, and pasta

Food names	Serving size	Fiber (grams)
100% bran cereal	1 oz.	8
Barley, cooked	1 cup	6.0
Whole-wheat spaghetti, cooked	1 cup	6.3
Buckwheat groats, cooked	1 cup	4.5
Bulghur, cooked	1 cup	8.2
Whole-wheat English muffins	1	4.4
Mixed grain bread	1 slice	2.1
Enriched spaghetti, cooked	1 cup	2.4
Wheat flakes	1oz.	3
Shredded wheat	1 biscuit	2
Oatmeal, instant	1 cup	4.0
Wheat bread (incl. wheat berry)	1 slice	1.1
Light rye bread	1 slice	1.9
Pumpernickel bread	1 slice	1.7
Enriched egg noodles, cooked	1 cup	1.8
Rye crispbread	1	1.6
Popcorn	2 cups	2
Brown rice, cooked	1 cup	3.5
Wild rice, cooked	1 cup	3.0
Bagel, oat bran	1	2.1
Rye wafers	1 cracker	2.5
Pasta	1/2 cup	1
Plain, enriched English muffin	1	1.5
Bagel, plain, enriched	1	1.3
Tortilla, corn	1 medium	1.4
White rice, cooked	1 cup	1
White bread	1 slice	1
Wheat dinner rolls	1-oz. roll	1
Breadsticks	1 small stick	1

Source: USDA database website

Vegetable group

Food names	Serving size	Fiber (grams)
Green beans, cooked	1 cup	8.8
Artichokes (globe, French), cooked	1	6.5
Baked potato skin	1	4.6
Baked potato, flesh	1	2.3
Green snap peas, cooked	1 cup	4.0
Broccoli, raw	1 cup flowerets	2.3
Cabbage, raw	1 cup	1.6
Bok choy, cooked	1 cup	2.7
Carrots, cooked	1/2 cup	2.6
Eggplant, cooked	1 cup	2.5
Lettuce, all varieties	1 cup	1
Shiitake mushrooms	1 cup	3.1
Onions, raw	1/2 cup	1.4
Pumpkin, cooked	1 cup	2.7
Spinach, cooked	1 cup	4.3
Zucchini, cooked	1 cup	2.9
Sweet potato, cooked, no skin	1 medium	2.7
Tomatoes, raw	1 cup	2.0
Watercress, raw	1 cup	4.6
Vegetable juice	1 cup	1

Source: USDA database website

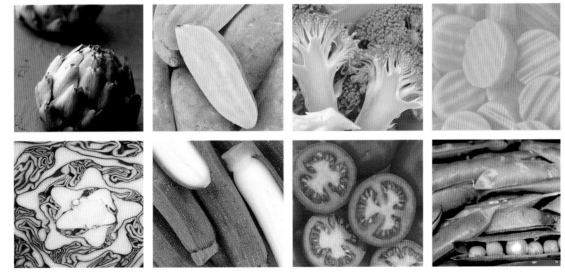

Fruit group

Food names	Serving size	Fiber (grams)
Apples, raw	1 cup	3.4
California avocado, raw	1	8.5
Florida avocado, raw	1	16.1
Banana	1 cup	3.6
Blueberries	1 pint	10.9
Cherries	1 cup	2.7
Cranberries, raw	1 cup	4.0
Dates, dried	1 cup	13.4
Grapefruit	1	2.5
Grapes, American	1 cup	0.9
Kiwi fruit	1	3.1
Mango	1	3.7
Melon, honeydew	1 cup	1.0
Oranges	1	3.6
Peach	1 large	3.1
Pear	1 medium	4.0
Pineapple	1 cup	1.9
Plums	1	1.0
Strawberries	1 cup	3.5
Watermelon	1 cup	1
Fruit juices	1 cup	1

Source: USDA database website

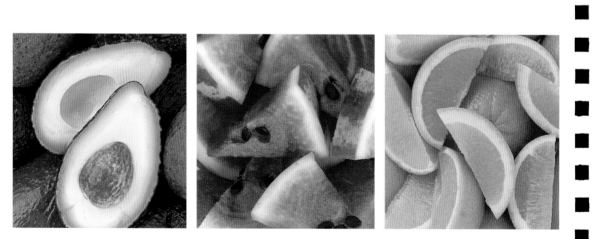

Meat, poultry, fish, dried beans, eggs, and nuts

Food names	Serving size	Fiber (grams)
Black beans, cooked	1 cup	15.0
Fava beans, cooked	1 cup	9.2
Chickpeas (garbanzo beans), canned	1 cup	10.6
Kidney beans, cooked	1 cup	11.3
Split peas, cooked	1 cup	16.3
Peanuts	1 oz.	2.3
Peanut butter, chunky	2 tbsp.	2.1
Soybeans, cooked	1 cup	10.3
Tofu, raw	1 cup	2.9

Source: USDA database website

pantry checklist: less is more

Next time you stock up on pantry basics, buy more wholegrain products. Use this list to help you choose the right foods.

Refined	More wholegrains
White bread	Whole-wheat bread
Bagels	Wholegrain bagels
Croissant	Wholegrain croissant
Muffins	Wholegrain oat or bran muffins
Flour tortillas	Corn or whole-wheat flour tortillas
Pasta	Whole-wheat, spinach, or corn pasta
Cookies	Oatmeal cookies
Cornflakes	Granola/bran flakes
Crackers	Graham crackers
White rice	Brown rice, red rice, wild rice
Rice noodles	Buckwheat or whole-wheat noodles
White flour	Replace a third in baked goods with whole-wheat flour or quick instant oats

expand your wholegrain repertoire

If you are bored of eating potatoes, pasta, and breads, you can easily expand your carb repertoire. Start your new regime by adding some of the wholegrains listed below to your daily diet:

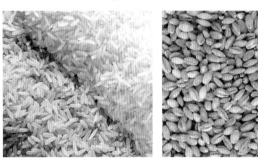

Barley This is low in fat and a great source of soluble fiber. It is also rich in protein, calcium, and potassium. Hulled barley has more fiber than quick-cook pearl barley.

Brown rice This has more fiber (four times more), vitamins, and minerals (including niacin, vitamin B6, magnesium, manganes, and phosphorous) than white rice because only the outer hull is removed during the processing. Brown rice is available in many varieties: long grain, medium grain, short grain, sweet rice, aromatic rice (for example, Thai Jasmine), and quick cook rice.

Buckwheat This is a grain that has been eaten for hundreds of years in the Far East, where it is roasted and ground into flour before being turned into noodles. Buckwheat can be used for a variety of baked products including pancakes, breads, muffins, crackers, bagels, cookies, and tortillas. Kasha, a traditional Jewish side dish, also uses buckwheat groats as its main ingredient. Buckwheat contains more protein than either wheat or oats.

Bulgur This is a processed form of whole-wheat. Whole-wheat kernels are steamed and dried, then cracked into pieces. It's easy to cook and only needs to be soaked in water

before it is used. It's a good source of complex carbs, insoluble fiber, protein, niacin, vitamin E, and minerals. Bulgur also contains lignans. These are phytochemicals and they are thought to help protect against developing heart disease.

Try to use the whole-wheat varieties of bulgur in order to gain its maximum benefits. It is available to buy in coarse, medium, or fine varieties. Coarse bulgur tends to be used for pilaf dishes, medium bulgur is often eaten like a cereal, and fine bulgur can be used as a replacement for couscous and also in stuffing, pilaf, soups, and casseroles.

Flaxseed This wholegrain contains an essential fatty acid called alpha-linolenic acid (ALA), which is converted by the body into a type of omega-3 fatty acids that has beneficial health properties. Omega-3 makes our blood cells less likely to stick together and they reduce blood clotting, thereby decreasing the risk of a heart attack.

Flaxseeds are the richest source of plant lignans and contain around 500 times more than wheat bran, rye, buckwheat, millet, soybeans, or oats. This grain is also a good source of insoluble fiber, as well as potassium. Unfortunately, some people are allergic to flaxseed and may go into anaphylactic shock if the reaction is severe. So be cautious when eating them for the first time or if you are cooking for other people.

To obtain its maximum health benefit, flaxseeds must be chewed well or ground before they are eaten (you can use a coffee grinder to do this but flaxseeds are available to buy ready-ground.) It is also available as an oil but it should be added to food only once it has been cooked as heating flaxseed makes it taste unpleasant. You can sprinkle ground flaxseeds onto your cereal, add them to the top of your muffin, bread, or cookie, or use them in your favorite smoothie.

Millet This grain is a rich source of B vitamins, phosphorous, zinc, copper, and soluble fiber.

Label Laws

Many manufacturers place fiber claims on their products. This is a summary of what is currently permitted by the U.S. Food and Drug Administration (FDA):

High fiber: This dictates that the food product should contain 5g or more of fiber per serving.

Source of fiber: This means that the product should have at least 2.5–4.9g of fiber per serving.

More or added fiber: This specifies that the product should contain at least 2.5g more per serving than the reference food.

One cup of cooked millet provides approximately 3.1g of fiber. Pearl millet can usually be bought from any good healthfood store and is pale yellow or orange in color.

It has a strong, nutty flavor and is relatively easy for our bodies to digest.

Quinoa An ancient Incan food, quinoa has more iron, calcium, B vitamins, copper, manganese, zinc, magnesium, and potassium than any other grain. But it actually isn't a grain at all—quinoa comes from the seed of a leafy plant related to spinach. It's a good substitute for rice, and you can use quinoa flour as a replacement for white flour in baked goods. The grains are small, about the same size as millet, and it cooks quickly, which makes it a great alternative to other grains. One cup of cooked quinoa contains 5g fiber.

Wild rice The name is misleading as this is not a true rice because it actually comes from the seed of a grass. Most wild rice is cultivated in paddies located in Northern California, Idaho, and Minnesota in the U.S. This type of rice contains more protein than white or brown rice and is a good source of potassium, zinc, folate, and fiber. It has a nutty flavor and can be used in salads, soups, breads, and stuffings.

carbs from fruit and vegetables

An ongoing study, started in 1993 by the European Prospective Investigation into Cancer and Nutrition (EPIC), has been following the diets of more than 400,000 people from nine countries. Preliminary results from this study reveal that an increase in a person's daily vitamin C intake (which can be as little as an extra apple a day or 2oz. of another fruit or vegetable) can cut the risk of dying early from any cause by 20 percent. Moreover, adding two additional servings of fruit and vegetables a day can reduce your risk by half.

If that wasn't a compelling enough reason for you to grab for the fruit bowl, then below is a list of some common fruit and vegetables and their additional health benefits.

Asparagus contains fructo-oligosaccharides (FOS) which promotes the growth of "good" bacteria in the gut. A study showed that volunteers taking a 4g daily supplement of FOS had an increased number of "good" bacteria called bifidobacteria in their gut and reduced levels of enzymes that promote cancer-causing compounds. Asparagus also contains phytochemicals

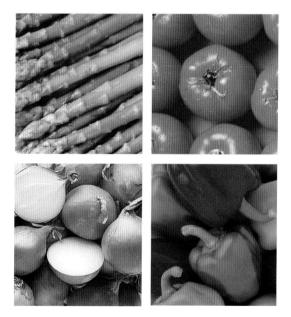

called saponins which have anticancer properties are also reputed to lower cholesterol.

Tomatoes are excellent sources of lycopene, especially ones that have been processed, for example canned tomatoes, tomato catsup, and tomato soup. Lycopene is a powerful antioxidant. A large study in the U.S. has shown that men who ate tomato products at least ten times a week had a 35 percent reduced risk of developing prostate cancer. Additionally, scientific studies have shown that lycopene is associated with a reduction in the risk of heart disease in men.

Onions are rich in flavonols called quercetin. Flavonols are potent antioxidants and studies in countries such as the U.S., Finland, and Greece have shown that quercetin has the ability to lower cholesterol as well as reducing the risk of heart disease. Onions contain high levels of compounds called allylic sulphides. These have the ability to induce enzymes that neutralize agents which cause cancer. In traditional chinese medicine, onions have been used to ease catarrh.

Bell peppers, particularly red and orange peppers, are rich in phytochemicals called beta-cryptoxanthin as well as beta-carotene. Research has shown that people with high levels of beta-cryptoxanthin have a reduced risk of angina. Bell peppers are also rich in capsaicin, a crystalline alkaloid which has been shown to have anti-inflammatory effects, (and which provides the "heat" in chiles) as well as aiding the digestive processes.

Spinach contains a phytochemical called lutein. Research has shown that lutein, in combination with the carotenoid zeaxanthin, protects against the development of age-related muscular degeneration (ARMD). ARMD is the most common cause of blindness in the Western world. Additional to this, a study in the U.S. has shown that eating lutein-rich foods may help to reduce the risk of developing cancer of the colon. Spinach is also rich in folate, which is beneficial as it reduces the risk of neural tube defects in unborn babies. In traditional chinese medicine spinach has been used as a treatment for constipation, high blood pressure, and anaemia.

Lettuce Different types of lettuce contain varying amounts of phytochemicals. For example, the lollo rosso variety is rich in flavonols, quercetin, lutein, and in the flavonoid anthocyanin, while romaine lettuce is an excellent source of zeaxanthin and lutein. Numerous studies have shown that quercetin and lutein can protect against cancer. A large study in the U.S. has shown that women who ate lettuce at least once a day had half the risk of breaking a hip than those who ate one or less portions of lettuce a week. In traditional chinese medicine, lettuce is thought to have sedative effects, therefore aiding a good night's sleep.

Carrots contain a phytochemical called beta-carotene which besides being a powerful antioxidant can also be converted into vitamin A in the body. It is true that carrots can help you see in the dark since a prolonged vitamin A deficiency can lead to night

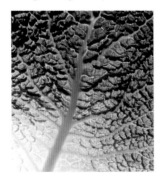

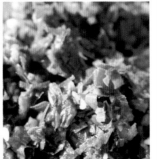

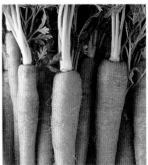

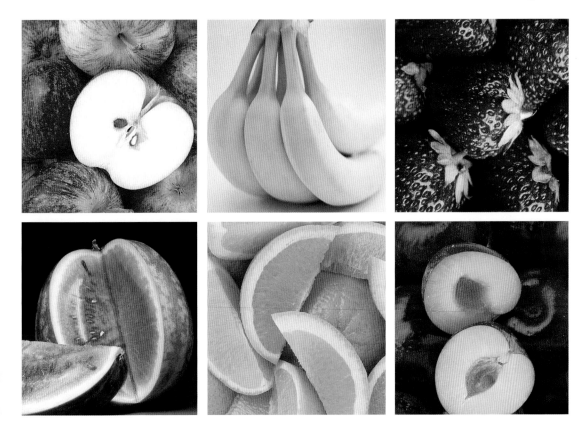

blindness. They may also help to reduce the risk of lung cancer. A long-term study in the U.S. on female nurses has shown that those who ate at least five carrots a week had a 60 percent lower risk of developing lung cancer than those who didn't eat any carrots at all.

Eggplant contains anthocyanins, particularly nasuin, which are potent antioxidants. Nasuin extracted from the skin of the eggplant has been shown in laboratory conditions to block the formation of free radicals. Free radicals are known to cause damage to cell membranes and the oxidation of "bad" LDL cholesterol, which can increase the risk of heart disease and strokes. In traditional chinese medicine, eggplant has been used to treat cancer and measles.

Cabbage contains phytochemicals called indoles. Indoles have been proven to have anticancer properties. Research on animals under laboratory conditions suggests that indoles may help fight cancer by stimulating the production of enzymes that form part of the body's detoxifying systems.

Broccoli contains the phytochemical sulphoraphane. Medical research has suggested that this particular chemical has the ability to block cancer-causing agents by stimulating the production of enzymes that form part of the body's detoxifying system. Studies have demonstrated that those people who have diets rich in cruciferous vegetables, like broccoli, have a reduced risk of developing cancer of the bowel, stomach, breast, lung, and kidney.

Apples contain flavonols called quercetin, which have been shown in numerous scientific investigations to possess anticancer properties. A long-term study, carried out in Finland, proved that eating lots of apples was strongly linked to a reduction in the risk of developing lung cancer. Quercetins have also been shown to exhibit anti-inflammatory properties and so they may well prove to be useful in the treatment of conditions such as arthritis. In traditional Chinese medicine, raw apples have historically been used to treat constipation, while cooked apples have been employed in the treatment of diarrhea.

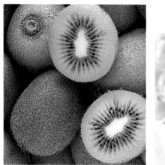 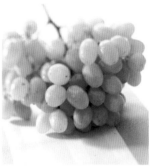 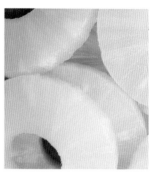

Strawberries contain ellagic acid which act as potent antioxidants and anticancer agents. Studies carried out under laboratory conditions have shown that ellagic acid can halt the growth of tumors in the lungs, esophagus, breast, cervix, and tongue. A study conducted in the U.S. also demonstrated that strawberries reduced the effects of carcinogens in tobacco smoke. In traditional chinese medicine, strawberries are thought to have antibacterial properties and were used to cleanse and detoxify the digestive system.

Bananas are an excellent source of vitamin B6. This vitamin is needed for our bodies to make a neurotransmitter, called serotonin, in the brain. Serotonin is known to reduce pain, depress the appetite, and make you feel relaxed and less stressed. In traditional chinese medicine, bananas have been used to treat stomach ulcers. Unlike other fruits, bananas are rich in carbohydrate.

Watermelons contain lycopene, which acts as a anticancer agent. Melons with red or orange flesh also contain carotenoids that, besides being able to protect body cells against damage from free radicals, can also be converted into vitamin A in the body. Vitamin A is required to maintain a healthy immune system, healthy skin, and good vision in dim light. Melons also have a high water content and one slice of watermelon is equivalent to a glass of water!

Oranges contain phytochemicals called hesperidin, which are powerful antioxidants that protect the body against damage from free radicals. They are also a good source of pectin, which can lower blood cholesterol.

Mangoes contain a carotenoid called beta-crytoxanthin which exhibit antioxidant properties and so may protect against some cancers such as colon and cervical cancer. A long-term study, which investigated the diets of a large group of women, showed that those eating a carotenoid-rich diet had a reduced risk of cervical cancer.

Kiwi fruit contains a pigment called chlorophyll, which gives the fruit its green color. Under laboratory conditions chlorophyll has been converted into compounds that have the ability to bind cancer-causing agents.

Plums contain a phytochemical called ferulic acid which has anticancer properties. More specific studies have shown that high intakes of ferulic acid are linked with a reduced risk of colonic cancer.

Grapes The skin of grapes contain a phytochemical called resveratrol, which has been proven to keep the heart healthy, and they also display anticancer, antibacterial, and antioxidant properties.

Pineapple contains the enzyme bromelain which has the ability to break down proteins. It is often used as a meat tenderizer. Bromelain nutritional supplements are available to buy and claims have been made that they are useful in relieving joint pain, helping with digestion, breaking up blood clots, combating sinusitis, and treating urinary tract infections.

Carbs: Friend or fiend?

Carbs

friend or fiend?

We now understand what carbs are and how they are broken down in the body. This section will now discuss why not all carbs are bad for us and why a moderate amount of carbs from our diet is important to our health.

As you know, carbohydrates have to be broken down during the process of digestion to create glucose. The energy we derive from glucose is the primary source of fuel for our body cells and if our supply of blood glucose becomes too low, we will can start to feel light headed, dizzy, or faint. When the body's glucose levels are depleted in this way it has to turn to other

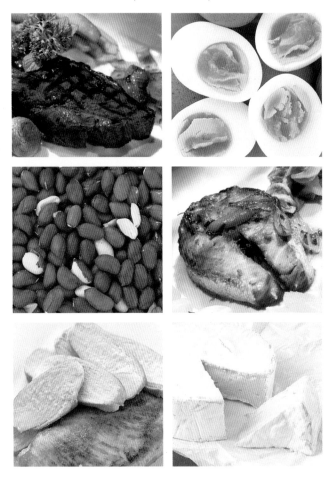

sources for fuel. This is when the importance of carbs in our diet becomes most apparent. When the body is deprived of glucose it will turn to protein for fuel, which means that the protein is no longer being used effectively. The carbs we normally consume prevent protein from being used as an energy source, but what is so important about protein that it has to be spared?

Well, the protein that comes from our diet, from meat, fish, nuts, beans, eggs, poultry etc., is needed to make body tissues and to perform other vital functions around the body, such as maintaining our immune system to help us fight infections and keeping us healthy. If you do not eat enough carbohydrates to make glucose, your body is forced into using the proteins stored in our cells. Proteins in our muscle cells are the first to be broken down to make glucose.

If the body continues to be starved of carbohydrates, the muscle cells will always progressively become weaker and weaker and vital tissues and organs, such as the heart, will eventually be affected.

Carbohydrates, however, do not simply act as an energy source. They have yet another important function because without them our body cannot handle fat in a "normal" way. This is because fat fragments have to be joined or combined with carbohydrates before they can be used for fuel. If fat is used for fuel without carbohydrates, the body is forced to go into a state called ketosis. This is when abnormal products called ketone bodies, resulting from the breakdown of fat, build up in our bloodstream.

The buildup of ketone bodies can have serious effects, particularly during pregnancy, as they can cause brain damage to the unborn

26

baby which can result in irreversible mental retardation after the baby is born.

So, to enable our body to make glucose and use fats as fuel in the normal way without jeopardizing the health of our immune system and other vital organs, a minimum amount of carbs—at least 50–100g—is needed every day to spare protein and to prevent ketosis. Health experts recommend an average of 200–400g of carbohydrates a day, or at least 55 percent of your total energy intake.

If you know your calorific intake, follow the math (right) to work out you ideal carb intake.

If you are consuming 2,000 calories a day, 55 percent of 2,000 calories would be:

$$\frac{55 \times 2000}{100} = \text{1,100 calories}$$

1g of carbohydrate yields 4 calories.
So, 1,100 calories would be equivalent to:

$$\frac{1100}{4} = \text{275g of carbohydrates a day}$$

what foods contain carbohydrates?

Almost all foods, apart from meat and fats, contain some carbohydrates. Let's look at the food pyramid in more detail.

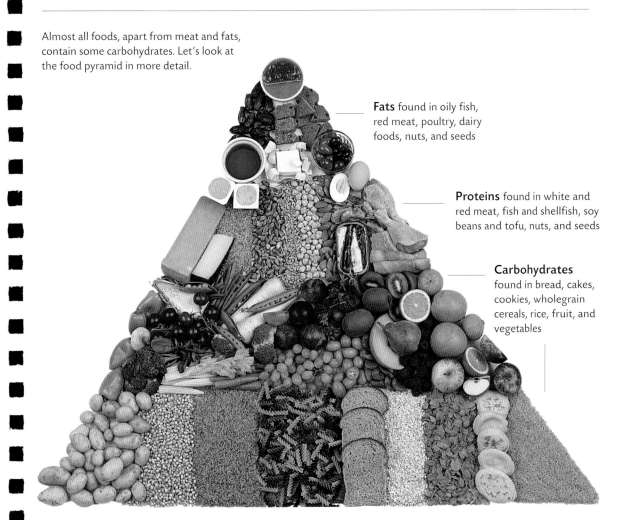

Fats found in oily fish, red meat, poultry, dairy foods, nuts, and seeds

Proteins found in white and red meat, fish and shellfish, soy beans and tofu, nuts, and seeds

Carbohydrates found in bread, cakes, cookies, wholegrain cereals, rice, fruit, and vegetables

Bottom tier: Bread, cereal, rice, and pasta

This group of grains includes bread, cereals, rice, and pasta and is the source of complex carbohydrates in your diet. These foods provide vitamins, minerals, fiber, and disease-fighting phytochemicals. In their natural state, complex carbohydrates are low in fat and low in calories provided you don't pile on mountains of butter and oil before you eat them! Remember that baked products like croissants, doughnuts, cookies, muffins, cakes, Danish, and other high fat and sugary foods belong to this group too, these are calorie dense and mostly refined and so should be kept to a minimum. The USDA's pyramid recommends that we should include between 6–11 servings of grains in our daily diet.

What is an average or medium serving?

People have different perceptions as to what constitutes a medium serving. Many snacks, restaurant meals, and take-out portions are much larger than the USDA size guide and seem to be increasing in size (and also in calories). A study published in 1998 compared what a group of students would consider as an average serving and the size recommended by the USDA pyramid. After a series of lectures on nutrition, students were asked to bring in at least one sample of what they considered to be a medium bagel, muffin, cookie, and potato. These were then weighed and compared with the reference weights. As you can see from the results below, the students' concept of a medium portion was at least double the reference serving size.

	Student's "medium" portion (oz.)	USDA "medium" portion (oz.)
Bagels	4.0	2.0
Muffins	5.5	1.5
Cookies	1.0	0.5
Baked potatoes	6.5	3.9

Take this short portion quiz to see how you are doing with your serving sizes:

1. What counts as a serving of bread?
a) $1/2$ slice
b) 1 slice
c) 2 slices

2. What is a serving of ready-to-eat cereal?
a) 1 oz.
b) 2 oz.
c) $1/2$ cup

3. What is a serving of cooked rice or pasta?
a) $1/2$ cup
b) 1 cup
c) 2 cups

4. One English muffin is equivalent to how many servings of grains?
a) 1
b) 2
c) 3

5. What is the correct serving size for a baked potato?
a) 1 small
b) 1 medium
c) 1 large

Correct Answers: 1. b. 2. a. 3. a. 4. b. 5. a

How did you do? No matter what your score was, I recommend that you use the guide opposite to help you choose your carbohyrdates servings for a balanced diet.

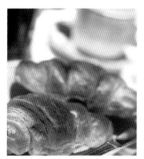
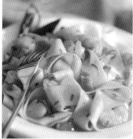
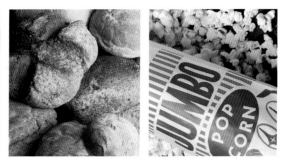

Listed below is a quick-reference guide to a few common food products that will help you determine what one serving of grains is equal to:

- 1 slice of bread
- half a hamburger or hot dog bun
- half an English muffin
- half a bagel
- 1 small muffin or cookie (1 oz.)
- 1 oz. ready-to-eat cereal
- 5–6 small saltine crackers
- 2–3 large Graham crackers
- 4 in. pita bread
- 3 medium hard breadsticks
- 1/2 cup cooked cereal
- 1/2 cup cooked rice or pasta
- one 7 in. flour or corn tortilla
- 2 corn taco shells
- 2 cups air popped popcorn
- 12 tortilla chips
- 1/16 of two-layer cake
- 9 animal crackers
- 1/2 cup uncooked rolled oats
- 3 tbsp. uncooked rice
- 9 three ring pretzels or 2 pretzel rods
- 1/5 of 10 in. angel food cake
- 1/10 of 8 in., two-crust pie
- 4 small cookies
- 1/2 large croissant
- 1/2 medium donut
- 3 rice cakes

Source: USDA

If you are still unsure about how many servings of grains you should be eating every day it will probably help if you are aware of how many calories you are recommended to consume on a daily basis. Listed here are the brief guidelines from the USDA on what level of calorie intake you should be on:

- 1,600 calories is about right for a woman who has a mainly sedentary lifestyle. At this level of intake you should aim to eat six servings of grains a day.
- 2,200 calories is about right for most children, teenage girls, active women*, and many sedentary men. Aim for nine servings of grains a day.
  Please note that pregnant or breastfeeding women may need more, so consult your doctor.
- 2,800 calories is about right for teenage boys, active men, and very active women. You should be eating around 11 servings of grains a day.

Remember to choose wholegrains wherever you can (refer back to Chapter 2 for detailed information on fiber). Here is a quick reminder of what foods are included in the category:

- Brown rice
- Buckwheat groats
- Bulgur
- Corn tortillas
- Graham crackers
- Granola
- Oatmeal
- Popcorn
- Ready-to-eat high fiber cereals
- Whole-wheat bread
- Whole-wheat rolls
- Whole-wheat crackers
- Whole-wheat pasta
- Whole-wheat cereals

Remember

Eating enriched foods is always preferable to consuming unenriched and refined, high-fat, high-sugar grain products.

Second tier: Fruit and vegetables

This group provides us with carbohydrates, vitamins, minerals, and fiber. The box below will tell you how many servings you need depending on your calorie intake. Then use the servings guide (below) to help you choose your two- to four-a-day fruit servings.

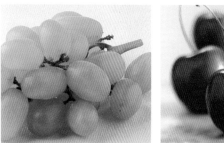
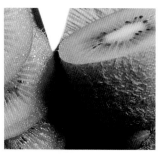
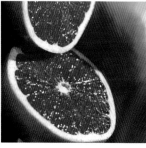

One serving of fruit is equal to:
- 1 medium whole apple or banana or peach or orange
- $1/2$ grapefruit
- $1/2$ of a medium cantaloupe or $1/8$ medium honeydew melon
- 7 melon balls
- $1/2$ cup 100% fruit juice
- $1/2$ cup cooked or canned fruit
- 5 large or 7 medium strawberries
- 12 grapes
- 11 large cherries
- 2 medium apricots

How Many Servings?

1,600 calories: aim for 2 servings of fruits
2,200 calories: aim for 3 servings of fruits
2,800 calories: aim for 4 servings of fruits

- 2 medium clementines
- $1/2$ cup fruit salad
- $1/2$ medium mango
- $1/2$ medium papaya
- 1 large kiwi fruit
- 2 canned pear halves with liquid
- $2^1/2$ slices canned pineapple halves with liquid
- $1/8$ medium avocado
- 50 blueberries
- 30 raspberries
- $1/2$ cup dried fruit
- 5 prunes
- 9 dried apricot halves

Source: USDA

Use this guide to help you with your three to five-a-day serving of vegetables:

One serving of $1/2$ cup cooked vegetables:
- 2 spears broccoli
- 1–$1^1/2$ whole carrots
- 1 medium whole green or red bell pepper
- $1/3$ yellow or green zucchini
- 1 globe artichoke
- 6 asparagus spears
- 2 whole beets
- 4 medium sprouts
- 2 medium stalks of celery
- 1 medium ear of corn
- 7 medium mushrooms
- 8 okra pods
- 1 medium onion or 6 pearl onions
- 1 medium whole turnip
- 10 French fries
- 1 medium baked potato
- $1/2$ cup sweet potato

One serving of $1/2$ cup raw vegetables:
- 1 medium tomato or 5 cherry tomatoes
- 1 cup mixed green salad
- $1/2$ cup coleslaw or potato salad
- 1 cup leafy vegetables such as kale or spinach or Swiss chard
- 7–8 carrot or celery sticks
- 3 broccoli florets
- $1/3$ medium cucumber
- 10 medium whole young green onions
- 8 green or red bell pepper rings

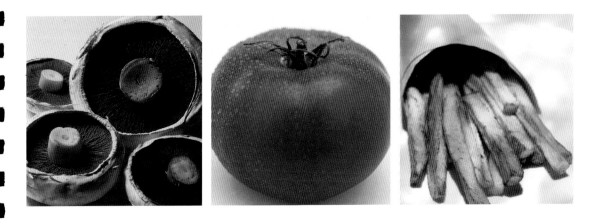

- 13 medium radishes
- 9 snow or sugar peas
- 6 slices of yellow or green zucchini
- $1/2$ cup tomato sauce
- $1/2$ cup tomato paste
- $1/2$ cup cooked dry beans
- $1/2$ cup vegetable juice
- 1 cup bean soup
- 1 cup vegetable soup

Source: USDA

Some vegetables contain more carbohydrates (or starch) than others. If you are trying to lose weight then you should limit your intake of starchy vegetables to one to two portions a day and choose the non-starchy vegetables. Examples of both are listed in the table below.

Starchy vegetables

beet greens, breadfruit, cassava, corn, green beans, hominy, lima beans, peas, potatoes, pumpkin, rutabago, sweet potatoes, taro, turnips, and yams

Non-starchy vegetables

asparagus, bok choy, broccoli, sprouts, cabbage, cauliflower, celery, chard, cucumber, eggplant, endive, green beans, kale, kohlrabi, romaine lettuce, mustard greens, mushroom, okra, bell peppers, radishes, tomatoes, and watercress

How Many Servings?

1,600 calories: aim for 3 servings of vegetables a day
2,200 calories: aim for 4 servings of vegetables a day
2,800 calories: aim for 5 servings of vegetables a day

Third tier: Meat and meat alternatives

Meat, fish, and poultry do not contain any carbs or fiber but good protein alternatives for this group, such as legumes (dry beans and peas), are great sources of complex carbs. Health experts recommend that you should eat two to three servings from this group a day.

One serving is equivalent to a 1 oz. or $1/3$ serving of the following foods:

- $1/2$ cup cooked dry beans
- 2 tbsp. peanut butter (*fat warning)
- $1/2$ cup sunflower or pumpkin seeds
- $1/3$ cup peanuts, walnuts, pistachio, or pecan nuts
- $1/2$ cup baked beans
- $1/2$ cup tofu

Source: USDA

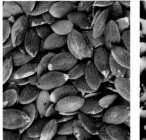
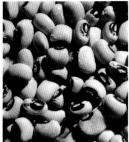

If you are confused about what legumes are, here is a short list of some of the most common dry peas and beans which you should be able to buy from most grocery stores:

- Black beans
- Black-eyed peas
- Chickpeas (garbanzo beans)
- Kidney beans
- Lentils
- Lima beans (mature)
- Mung beans
- Navy beans
- Pinto beans
- Split peas

Fourth tier: Dairy products

This group includes milk, yogurt, and cheese and is a source of vitamins, minerals, and milk sugar. Health experts recommend two servings (three for pregnant or breastfeeding mums, teenagers, and young adults) whatever daily calorie level you are on.

One serving of dairy produce is equivalent to:

- 1 cup milk (skim, low-fat, whole)
- 1 cup or 8 oz. yogurt (all kinds)
- 1–1 $\frac{1}{2}$ oz. natural cheese, for example, 2 cups cottage cheese or $\frac{1}{2}$ cup ricotta cheese
- 2 oz. process cheese
- 1–1 $\frac{1}{2}$ cups ice cream

Source: USDA

Remember to always choose lower fat versions of any of these products if you are watching your weight. Here is a quick reminder:

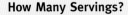

How Many Servings?

1,600 calories:
Aim for 5 oz. of dairy produce a day
2,200 calories:
Aim for 6 oz. of dairy produce a day
2,800 calories:
Aim for 7 oz. of dairy produce a day

- Low-fat buttermilk
- Low-fat cottage cheese
- Low-fat milk (1% and 2% fat)
- Low-fat unflavored yogurt
- Non-fat unflavored yogurt
- Skim milk

Source: USDA

Although it is recommended we eat a certain amount of dairy produce a day in order to achieve a healthy, balanced diet, there are some dairy products that are definitely diet saboteurs. You should always limit your intake of the following foods, as they are high in sugar and fat:

- Cheddar cheese
- Flavored or chocolate milk
- Flavored yogurt
- Frozen yogurt
- Fruit yogurt
- Ice cream
- Processed cheese
- Processed cheese spreads
- Milk puddings, for example, crème caramel, custard, trifles, chocolate pudding
- Whole milk

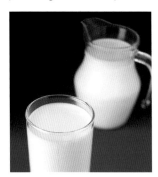
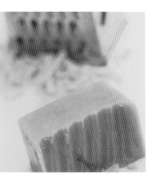
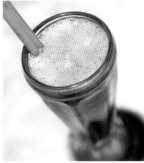

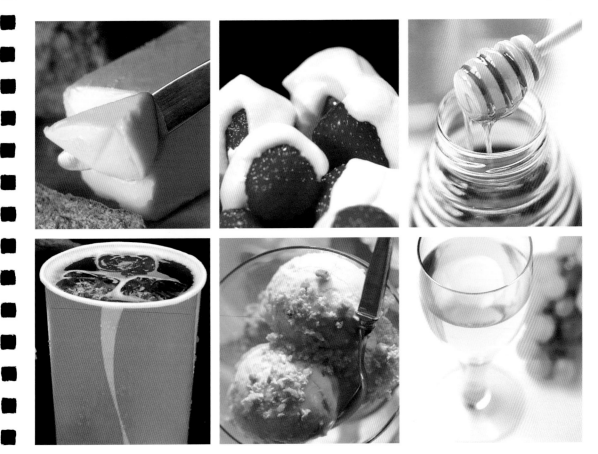

Portions At A Glance

Confused by cup sizes? Can't tell what is an ounce without taking out your weighing scales? Then use the following guide from the American Dietetic Association, based on a the size of a woman's hand to help you:

- 1 cupped hand is equivalent to a 3 oz. serving of nuts or small candies
- 1 cupped hand is equivalent to $1/2$ oz. serving of chips, popcorn, or pretzels
- Tip of the thumb is equivalent to 1 tsp.
- 1 thumb is equivalent to 1 tbsp. of liquid
- 1 thumb is equivalent to 1 oz. of cheese
- 1 fist is equivalent to 1 cup of ice cream or frozen yogurt
- 1 fist is equivalent to 1 cup of cereal, pasta, rice
- 1 fist is equivalent to 1 cup of fruit or vegetables

Fifth tier: Fats, candy, and alcoholic beverages

Go easy on foods from this group. Desserts, candy, and alcoholic beverages all contain simple carbs. Although fats like butter, cream, and cream cheese contain milk sugar, they are all calorie-dense and so should be limited.

Here's the hit list:
- Butter
- Cream
- Lard/shortening
- Cream cheese
- Mayo
- Sour cream
- Candy
- Frosting
- Corn syrup
- Honey
- Fruit drinks
- Jelly
- Jello
- Marmalade
- Maple syrup
- Molasses
- Table sugar
- Ice cream
- Sodas
- Colas
- Sugar
- Beer
- Liquor
- Wine

Source: USDA

33

do you turn to carbs for comfort?

To discover whether you are taking comfort from carbs answer the following questions truthfully. Remember, there is no point in lying to yourself—and there is no one else listening in.

1. Is your pantry stocked with bags of supersize candy, cookies, chips, chocolate, or donuts and/or is your freezer bursting with ice cream and frozen desserts?
Yes or No

2. Do you snack on sweet or starchy foods at least once a day?
Yes or No

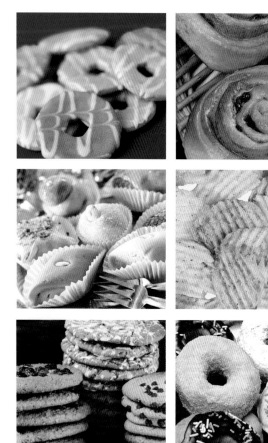

3. Do you head to the fridge freezer or pantry when you are bored?
Yes or No

4. Do you regularly snack on sweet or starchy foods when you are watching the television even if you have just eaten dinner?
Yes or No

5. Do you head to the refrigerator or pantry when you can't sleep?
Yes or No

6. Do you head to the refrigerator or pantry if you have had a rough day at home or work?
Yes or No

7. Do you head to the refrigerator, freezer, or pantry when you have had an argument with your partner, parents/in-laws, kids, etc.?
Yes or No

If you have answered yes to more than two of these questions, then you could be an emotional carbophile.

We often turn to candy, cookies, chips, etc., in stressful situations because we think that it makes us feel calmer and tranquil. Perhaps it's all to do with conditioning early on in our childhood or it could be something to do with gender.

Interestingly, some studies have shown that men in stressful situations turn to comforting dishes such as chicken soup or homemade casseroles that they remember their mom used to make while women regularly turn to chocolate or ice cream to cheer them up.

So, why do most people turn to carbs for comfort? Well, remember in the earlier chapters that carbohydrate-rich foods such as rice, pasta, potatoes, cereals, noodles, yam, and bread have the ability to trigger the release of a hormone called insulin into the blood stream. This is important as insulin, besides being able to shunt excess glucose into our fat cells, also has the ability to promote the uptake of amino acids (building blocks for protein) into body cells with the exception of tryptophan. With the other amino acids cleared from the bloodstream, tryptophan enters the brain unimpeded, there it is converted into a neurotransmitter called serotonin which has the effect of elevating mood, suppressing appetite, reducing pain, inducing sleep, and promoting a feeling of calmness.

Low levels of serotonin can contribute to the clinical depression of some depressed patients. Some anti-depressant medications are designed to make serotonin more active in the brain for longer periods of time to help regulate mood.

According to research at the Massachusetts Institute of Technology Clinical Research Center in Boston, U.S., some people can be classified as carbohydrates cravers. They tend to experience a change in their mood usually in the late afternoon or early evening and long to eat something sweet or starchy. If they fill up with protein instead then this group of people become grumpy and irritable. Sufferers from a form of depression called seasonal affective disorder (or SAD) also tend to crave carbohydrates when they are depressed.

So that's why you feel that an entire packet of cookies or a supersize bag of chips will make you feel better! It probably does—in the short term.

will I stay an emotional carbophile for ever?

Use a diary, like the one on the next page, for the next two weeks to write down all of the triggering factors that make you crave carbs (for example, anger, tiredness, depression, or frustration). Note down whether you were actually hungry when you decided to binge on that candy bar. Where were you watching the TV, preparing dinner, surfing the net, or helping your kids with homework? At the end of the two weeks, look at your diary and you will be able see a pattern that you can now work positively toward to control your carb cravings.

If stress is the predominant factor, then every time you reach for the cookies, make a conscious effect to put them back and do something else that calms you down. It can be anything from having a long soak in the bath, taking the dog out for a walk, phoning a friend for a chat,

or reading your favorite magazine, so long as it works for you. Similarly, if the triggering factor is the TV, make a conscious effort to break your carb cravings. Try swapping your bag of candied popcorn for a piece of fruit or switching off the TV and doing something else that involves some exercise. For example, put a favorite CD on and dance along with the music.

If the triggering factor is because you were too busy and skipped lunch, then make a special effort to make some time-out for yourself. Experiment with the recipes in the back of this book, perhaps you could make a comforting soup, easy salad, or bread, and enjoy the process of making time to provide nourishment for yourself. Inviting someone to share a meal would be a great reward and would help you to unwind.

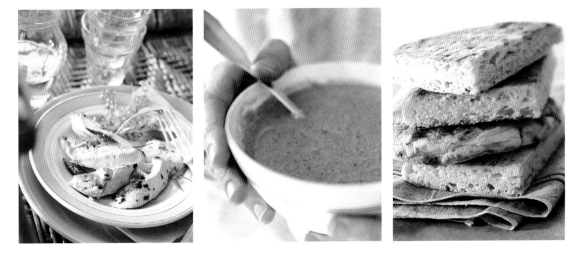

Comfort eating diary

Day	Situation	Mood	Place	Food
1. Monday	Fight with partner over breakfast	Frustrated and angry	Kitchen	3 Donuts
2. Tuesday	Worked overtime	Felt I deserved a reward	Candy machine	Snickers bar
3.				
4.				
5.				
6.				
7.				
8.				
9.				
10.				
11.				
12.				
13.				
14.				

Are all carbs equal?

Are all carbs equal?

slow and fast glucose release

We need carbohydrates in our diet to provide our body with an accessible and immediate energy source and to prevent ketosis. But are all carbs good for us?

Are the carbs found in cookies and donuts the same carbs from pumpernickel bread or whole-wheat cereals? The answer to this is no and there is a simple system that can help us to understand the differences between them—the GI. No, I am not referring *those* men in uniform, but the next best thing since the invention of sliced bread, the Glycemic Index.

what is the glycemic index?

As we have already learnt from the earlier chapters in this book, energy is needed to perform the various basic functions in the body, whether it is maintaining our heart beat, walking, runnning, thinking, or simply keeping our bodies ticking over while we sleep. We know that the body's preferred fuel is glucose, which is supplied by simple sugars and by the digestion of starchy foods like rice, cereals, potatoes, pasta, breads, legumes, and some fruits and vegetables.

The rates at which different types of food is broken down during digestion vary greatly. Some foods are converted rapidly into glucose. These are labeled as high glycemic index foods and include most types of simple carbs. Other foods are broken down more slowly and are referred to as low glycemic index foods. They include most types of complex carbs.

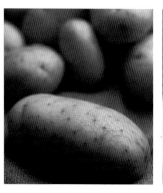 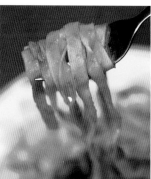

The Glycemic Index was originally developed as a research tool to rank foods according to the rate at which it raises our blood sugar levels relative to pure glucose. The rate at which pure glucose raises our blood sugar is used as the standard measurement and is assigned a GI score of 100. So the closer to 100 a particular food is, the higher its glycemic index ranking.

The good carb/bad carb theory

Up until the early 1980s, scientists thought that simple carbohydrates (such as those provided by sugars, candy, cookies, preserves, etc.) produce swifter rises in blood sugar than complex carbohydrates (from foods such as breads, rice, potatoes, legumes, fruits, vegetables, etc.).

However, recent research has turned this theory on its head. A number of starchy foods such as carrots, mashed potatoes, some types of rice, and breads are in fact digested and absorbed far more rapidly causing blood sugar levels to spike, while candy, some cookies, and cakes actually have a lower GI than bread!

The rise and fall of glucose

Some of us love the thrills of a rollercoaster, but our bodies prefer to remain at an even keel and maintain a strict regulatory system to avoid major swings in our blood sugar levels.

When glucose is released into the bloodstream during digestion, the body produces a storage hormone called insulin whose job it is to carry the glucose to places where it is needed for fuel—primarily to the brain and muscle cells. While our bodies can deal with a steady release of glucose during digestion, when large amounts enter the bloodstream our regulatory system starts to work in overdrive and produces large quantities of insulin to clear the glucose away.

Perversely, these surges of insulin actually increase our feelings of hunger and, in a vicious circle, increases our desire to eat more simple carbs. This works to our detriment since any excess glucose we consume is transported to our fat cells where it can be stored in unlimited amounts! If this happens frequently it can obviously lead to weight gain, but more importantly it can damage our cells by causing insulin resistance. This damage can then result in premature aging, furring up of the arteries, and it may even trigger Type II or middle-aged onset diabetes.

the GI way of eating

There are many versions of this way of eating, but the underlying principle of all of them is that you have to base your diet on foods that have a low GI score. In other words, these diet plans encourage you to eat foods that cause a steady rise in blood sugar and advise you to limit those which have a medium to high GI. Some foods that don't contain starchy carbs do not have a GI score and can be eaten freely. For example water, coffee, oil, most fruits and vegetables, and protein-rich foods such as meat, fish, eggs, duck, and seafood are all acceptable.

There are many factors that can influence the GI count of a food, and below are listed some of these variables:

- The smaller the particle size, the higher the GI. So, the more processed the food the higher the GI. For example, cornflakes have a higher GI than muesli.
- Fat slows down the rate of digestion and so lowers the GI score of a food. For example, French fries have a lower GI than boiled or mashed potatoes.
- Soluble fiber from beans, pulses, legumes, fruits, and oats slows down the rate of digestion and so these foods have lower GIs.
- Protein slows down the rate at which carbohydrates are digested and so lowers the overall GI of a food or meal. For example, eating meat or poultry with boiled rice or potatoes will lower their GI.
- Two types of starch exist in foods: amylose and amylopectin. Amylose' structure is long and straight and so it's difficult for enzymes to break it down, while amylopectin's structure is branched and so makes it easier for enzymes to digest. Therefore, the more amylose a food contains, the longer it takes the body to digest it, and the lower the GI. For example, pulses and legumes have a higher amylose content and therefore a lower GI, while wheat flour and foods that contain wheat flour have a higher GI.
- The type of sugar a food contains will also vary its GI count. Pure glucose raises blood sugar levels rapidly. However, fructose (fruit sugar) is converted to glucose slowly, as is lactose (milk sugar) and therefore foods containing these types of sugars have a lower GI.
- Acidity slows down digestion and so lowers the GI of a food. For example, citrus fruits, the presence of vinegar, or lactic acid (in milk products) in food, all lower the GI score of any particular food.

A typical day's menu on a GI diet plan

Breakfast: Granola, slice of whole-wheat stoneground toast, an orange, coffee, a glass of non-fat milk.

Lunch: Chicken, argula, and roasted bell pepper with whole-wheat pasta.

Dinner: White bean soup, broiled salmon with pesto, broiled asparagus, and either new potatoes or basmati rice. Berry crumble (with oats and whole-wheat flour).

Snacks allowed: Apple and bran muffins, low-fat cottage cheese with fruit, and raw vegetables with red bell pepper, hummus.

Source: Rick Gallop (2003) The G.I. Diet: The Easy Healthy Way to Permanent Weight Loss. Workman publishing

Tables 1–3 on the following pages provide you with a simple reference guide to those foods with high, medium, and low GI counts:

Data from www.glycemicindex.com

The Scoring System

- Low = 0–39
- Medium = 40–59
- High = 60–100

1. High Glycemic Index foods

Foods	Glycemic Index	Serving size (grams)
White bread	69–87	30
Bagels	72	70
Baguette	95	30
Instant oatmeal	66	250
Quick-cook (instant) rice	87–94	150
Mashed potatoes	67–83	150
Instant mashed potatoes	87–94	150
Donuts	76	47
Flaked cereals (cornflakes, wheat flakes, bran flakes)	74–92	30
Sticky jasmine rice	109	150
Hard candy	80–101	30
Puffed rice cakes	87	25
Watermelon without seeds	80	195
Dates	103	60
Parsnips	97	80
Pumpkin	75	80
Popcorn	89	20
Rutabaga	72	150
Fava beans	79	80
French fries (microwaveable)	75	150
Sport drinks	95	269
Sodas	84	262

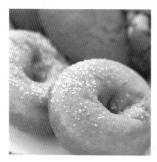
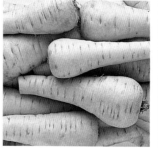
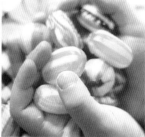

2. Medium Glycemic Index foods

Foods	Glycemic Index	Serving size (grams)
Pita bread	57	30
Wild rice	57	150
Basmati rice	58	150
Couscous	61	150
Baked potatoes (Canadian Pontiac, Russet Burbank varieties)	55–56	150
Granola (Swiss type)	56	30
Udon noodles	62	180
Potato chips	57	50
Bananas (not South African)	58	120
Papaya	56–60	120
Beets	64	80
Orange juice	57	264
Cranberry juice drink	56	253
Soda	63	261
Fruit concentrates	66	255

Health experts believe that the GI way of eating can have some advantages for diabetic patients and those watching their waistlines. The diet plan works simply because you will learn more about the different kinds of carbohydrates you eat. You are encouraged to eat more complex carbohydrates than simple, refined ones, which should help you to become a healthier eater. Plus, because eating complex carbohydrates delays the feeling of hunger, compared to eating simple carbohydrates, it can also help you control your calorie intake, too. The glycemic index concept may be especially useful for diabetic patients who are required to carefully control their blood sugar levels, as eating low GI foods means glucose is released slowly into the bloodstream. (See Chapter 9 for further discussion of special diets).

How do you work out the GI of a meal?

Since we usually eat combinations of foods rather than single foods, you may wonder what how useful the GI is as it only gives you the score for individual foods. However, it is possible to make an approximate estimate of the GI of a simple meal. For example, if you had roughly equal portions of two foods, you simply add the GI values together and divide by two. Below are two examples of how to calculate this.

Yogurt and apple snack
The GI of yogurt is 33
The GI of apple is 38

The GI of this snack meal is:

$$\frac{33+38}{2} = 36$$

Baked beans and potato
GI of baked beans is 48
GI of baked potato is 85

The GI of this meal is:

$$\frac{38+85}{2} = 67$$

41

3. Low Glycemic Index foods

Foods	Glycemic Index	Serving size (grams)
Barley kernel bread	34	30
Pumpernickel bread with wholegrains	41	30
Soya and linseed bread	36	30
Bran strands	30–50	30
Barley kernel bread	27	30
Sourdough bread	54–55	30
Wheat tortillas	30	62
Buckwheat	46	150
Bulghur wheat	46	150
Barley	22	150
New potatoes	47	150
Mung bean noodles	25	150
Yam	25–34	150
Brown rice (USA)	50	150
Sweet potatoes (Australia and Canada)	44–48	150
Pasta (all types)	43–54	180
Chocolate (semisweet and bittersweet)	42–45	50
Yoghurt (low-fat and no-fat)	14–28	200
Ice cream (low-fat)	37–38	50
Milk	21	258
Peanuts	7–23	50
Cashew nuts	22	50
Mango (Phillipines and Australia)	41–51	120
Grapes	43–49	120
Corn on the cob and sweetcorn kernels	48	50
Apples	32–44	120
Strawberries	40	120
Orange	31–51	120
Grapefruit	25	120
Lentils (not canned)	18–32	150
Butter beans	29	150
Chickpeas (garbanzo beans)	10	150
Kidney beans	25	150
White beans	13	150
Mung beans	31	150
Split peas	32	150
Tomato juice	38	257
Vegetable juice	43	163

pros and cons of the GI

The pros: Benefits for health and weight loss

- You are less likely to feel hungry after a low GI meal. Most low GI foods are high in fiber and protein, which tend to fill you up for longer. They slow down the absorption of carbohydrate and therefore the rate at which glucose is released into the bloodstream.
- A slower release of glucose into the bloodstream means that smaller quantities of insulin are produced and therefore excess glucose will not be pushed into our fat stores.
- Glucose causes the release of insulin, which is an appetite stimulant. Therefore less glucose equals less insulin, which means you are likely to want to eat less.
- As less insulin is produced, the body releases another hormone called glucagon into the bloodstream. Glucagon has the function of taking glucose out of fat cells to be used as fuel.

The cons: Potential pitfalls with weight loss

- Individual metabolic differences, different cooking methods, whether the food is eaten cooked or raw or in a different form, and what other foods are eaten with the food in question, all affect the GI of the food. Since the GI is calculated on an individual food basis, it cannot be easily applied to foods when eaten in combinations, which is what we usually do.
- The plan does not mention anything about controlling your portions. Remember portions are often super-sized, many offers of B.O.G.O.F. (buy one get one free) tempting us into eating more than we want or need, which means we consume more calories. Remember that just because a food has a low GI does not mean it should be eaten in unlimited amounts.
- Some very healthy food choices, such as raw carrots and mashed potatoes have relatively high GI!

smart eating

Below are some points to remember if you are following the GI concept:
- Although the GI is useful to know about, it should not be the only guide you adhere to, and is best followed in the context of the Healthy Diet Food Pyramid (see Chapter 2).
- High GI foods are not all "bad" and similarly, low GI foods are not all "good." For example, for an athlete needing to replenish their glycogen (carbohydrate) stores after training, high GI foods are ideal (see Chapter 6 for further discussion on carbs and sport). While an energy-dense food with a low GI is not necessarily ideal for those watching their weight.

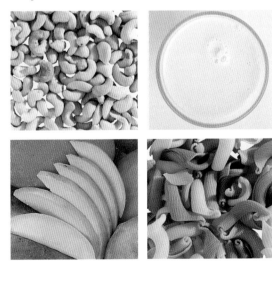

Here are some top tips for successful GI eating:
- Watch your portion sizes.
- Keep fatty and sugary foods to a minimum, and make sure you choose low-fat and reduced-sugar versions wherever possible, even though some of these foods may have a high GI score.
- Choose to snack on fruits and vegetables. Most have a low GI score.
- Go vegetarian once in a while or make your dishes go further by adding pulses and beans to increase the fiber content.
- Eat wholegrain breads, wholegrain cereals, and brown rice rather than their processed and refined cousins.
- Choose low to moderate GI foods whenever you can.
- Finally, if you are eating a high GI food, eat at least a couple of larger servings of low GI foods at the same time to balance out the overall GI score of your meal.

resolve to eat healthier carbs

Use the following resolutions to help you eat healthier carbs during the next two weeks:

Day 1: I must grab two pieces of fruit on my way back from picking up the children from school and snack on them before dinner tonight.

Day 2: I must try a fruit smoothie with non-fat milk as a mid-morning snack to boost my fiber and energy levels.

Day 3: I must swap my usual packet of potato chips for a handful of air popped popcorn today.

Day 4: I will eat my bran cereal this morning, and top it up with fresh fruit instead of buying a waffle or donut on my way to work.

Day 5: I will tidy up my pantry and throw away any cookies, candy, or cakes I find so I will not be tempted to snack on them.

Day 6: I will buy smaller servings of my favorite high-fat, high-sugar foods; otherwise I will find it difficult to stop eating even when I am full.

Day 7: I will not pile any butter onto my baked potato for dinner.

Day 7: I will include some leeks or cabbage tonight for dinner because they are high in fiber and contain phytochemicals that will help to keep me healthy.

Day 8: I will include more vegetables, beans, and pulses in the casserole that I am going to cook tonight because these provide great sources of protein and fiber and are virtually fat-free.

Day 9: I will wake up earlier so that I can eat breakfast this morning. Instead of sprinkling sugar on my cereal, I will add dried fruit or ground cinnamon instead. I might even make some oatmeal and serve it with dried dates and cinnamon.

Day 10: From today I will not eat my children's leftovers.

Day 11: I will try not to eat too late tonight because I will be really hungry and tired and that makes me want to overeat.

Day 12: Instead of eating spaghetti tonight I will try some Quinoa or red rice; these have more fiber in them and will add more variety to my diet.

Day 13: I will try to control the amount of food I eat by serving it on a smaller plate. When I eat out, I will make a conscious effort to leave some food behind on my plate.

Day 14: I will buy a juicer and start making delicious vegetable and fruit juices, and smoothies. In this way I am sure to meet all my daily requirements for essential vitamins, minerals, and phytochemicals with very little extra effort.

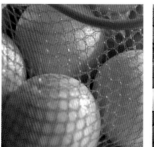 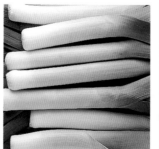 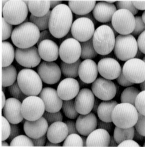

Simple or complex carbs?

Simple or complex carbs

which is better?

As you now know, not all carbs are equal. Simple carbs are easier for our body to digest and are absorbed quickly into the bloodstream, whereas complex carbs take a lot longer to break down and are absorbed more slowly.

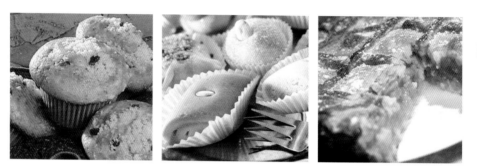

sugar on trial

Simple carbs, such as sugar, constantly receive a bad press and are blamed for causing obesity, diabetes, heart disease, hyperactivity in children, and dental decay. So, has the accused been found guilty on all counts or is the jury still out? Let's look at the evidence.

Background

Health experts recommend that simple sugars added to foods should not provide more than 10 percent of our total energy intake. So, if your recommended daily calorie intake is 2,000 calories, you shouldn't be consuming more than 50g or 10 teaspoons of simple sugars a day. Unfortunately, many of us eat much more than this and most of the sugars we eat come from foods and drinks that have had sugar added to them during processing. Here is a list of some of the guilty items:

• Candy
• Muffins
• Cakes
• Cookies
• Pies
• Ice cream
• Desserts
• Donuts
• Sodas
• Fruit drinks, fruit cocktail, and fruitades
• Sugar-coated cereals
• Added sugar (added by us!)

Foods with a high added sugar content have a high glycemic index (refer back to Chapter 4 for details) and these increase the production

Added & Naturally Occuring

Sugars added to foods to increase sweetness or bulk are termed "added" sugars. Sugars that are present naturally, like those in fruit and milk, are referred to as "naturally occurring" sugars. Start believing that Nature is sweet enough!

of insulin. A chronic increase can have disastrous effects on the body leading to any number of the following:

- High blood triglycerides (fat).
- An increase in smaller, low-density lipoprotein (LDL) particles, which raise the risk of heart disease.
- Increased deposits of fat in fat cells.
- Increased tendency for the blood to clot.

- Increased production of fat from the liver cells.

Finally, a rise in the production of insulin makes you feel hungry much more quickly after a meal. If this increased production of insulin continues over a long period of time, muscle cells will become resistant to insulin, which may eventually lead to diabetes for some people (see Chapter 9 for details on special diets).

sugar and obesity

Obesity is one of the fastest growing health problems in the world. The World Health Organization is treating it as an epidemic—serious words from a serious source. Between the late 1980s and early 1990s, the prevalence rate of obesity was 22.9 percent in the U.S. In 2000, this had increased to 30.5 percent. One-third of adults in the U.S. are now considered obese and two-thirds as overweight. Over the same period, in the U.K. eight percent of women and six percent of men were registered as obese. By 1998, the figures had increased to 21 percent of women and 17 percent of men.

For many years, cutting down on fat has been the focus of those of us wanting to lose weight. Recently attention has been shifting onto sugars and their role in the obesity epidemic. Some foods that are low in fat are high in added sugars and so actually provide similar calories to those that have a regular fat content. Most added sugars are simple carbs and come from candy, confectionery, and sodas.

An article in the *Journal of Pediatrics*, published in 2003, suggests that the increase in consumption of sugary sodas may be stoking the rise in obesity. Studies published in the *American Journal of Clinical Nutrition* between 1990 and 2002 support this statement. Their investigations showed that volunteers who were given sugar-rich, artificially sweetened drinks, rather than water, at a meal still ate the same amount of foods, making no compensation for the calories the drinks provided. The obvious result of the study was that the group consuming sugar-rich drinks took in more calories

than the other group. Interestingly, researchers at the Pennsylvania State University found that healthy women instinctively eat around three pounds (1.35 kg) of food a day and it did not matter whether it was high or low in calories. Therefore, their conclusion was that it is volume, rather than calories, that drives us to eat.

The moral of both stories is plain: simple carbs from concentrated sweets, sugary drinks, preserves, and other confectionery make it easy for us to eat large amounts of calories quickly and conveniently. These refined foods are low in fiber while being calorie-dense and so we want to eat more because we do not feel full up.

The result is that we eat far more calories than we actually need and together with our increasingly sedentary lifestyles this means that many of us take in more energy than we expend. That extra energy, as we all know, goes towards an unlimited store of fat which is unhealthy and—over long periods of time—potentially life threatening.

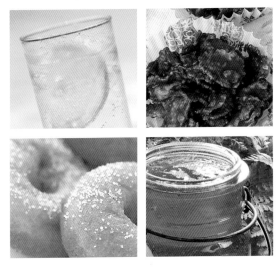

Did You Know?

The sugar content of a food is often increased after processing. The more processed the food, the higher the sugar content.

sugar and dental decay

Dentists and health experts now all agree that sugars and starches which are readily fermented in the mouth—such as those from white bread, chips, and crackers—increase the risk of developing dental caries or tooth decay.

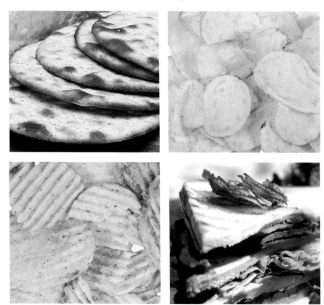

sticky substance that needs to be scraped off our teeth every time we visit the dental hygienist. Plaque not only helps bacteria stick to our teeth but they also diminish the acid neutralizing effect of our saliva. Sucrose, or regular sugar, is the most common offender when it comes to dental caries although glucose, maltose, and sticky foods, like caramel, are also cariogenic (*cario* = cavities, *genic* = producing) and are equally likely to cause caries.

It appears that the amount of sugar consumed at any one time is less important than how often sugar-containing foods and drinks are consumed. That means that snacking frequently on sugary foods gives the bacteria on our teeth a steady supply of simple carbs from which to produce acids.

So the message is simple: eating less sugary foods and drinks gives our teeth a chance to repair themselves between meals. Health experts have suggested that limiting sugar-containing food and drink to meal times is one way to help us to reduce the incidence of caries.

How does this happen?
Caries form when sugars (and other carbs) are changed into acids by bacteria that live in our mouth. These acids dissolve the tooth enamel and the structures that lie underneath. Sugars are also used by bacteria to create plaque—the

Tip
Cheese, peanuts, and sugar-free chewing gum reduce the amount of acid on our teeth, as does rinsing the mouth after meals and snacks.

sugar and hyperactivity

Children can often become over-excited, energetic, excitable, restless, irritable, disruptive, or even aggressive after mealtimes or snacks. Many people attribute this to children being allowed to eat too many sugary foods, food additives, or caffeine. But is the association between sugary foods and hyperactivity in children a justified assumption?

What is hyperactivity ?
Hyperactivity is characterized by symptoms such as restlessness, irritability, aggressiveness, and short attention span. Some studies have reported that around 5–10 percent of children are actually hyperactive. The possible link between sugary foods and such behavior was first hypothesized in the early 1920s when hyperactivity was thought to be a result of an

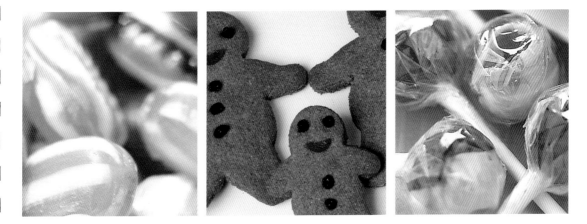

allergic response to refined sugar—back then it was labeled as tension fatigue syndrome. Today many theories exist about the links between sugar and behavior. The following is a brief summary of just some of them:

Behavioral changes and sugar
Some researchers believe that behavioral changes may occur as a result of a series of hormones being released after consuming sugar. One of these hormones is norepinephrine, otherwise known as stress hormone. This theory was tested in a study looking at the norepinephrine levels among a small group of adults and children after they had been given a sugar-rich drink. The study found that the resultant norepinephrine levels measured in the children were double the amount found in the adults.

The Halloween effect
Quite simply, the theory is that because sugar provides energy it therefore affects behavior. This theory was tested in a small study group of children who had been hospitalized for psychiatric disorders. Children were either given pure orange juice or orange juice to which fructose and sucrose had been added. The study showed that children given the juice with added sugars became more active and displayed more inappropriate behavior than the control group. The theory is that the added calories allowed the children to exert more energy.

The calming effect of sugar
Several recent studies have demonstrated that rather than triggering restlessness, sugar tended to exert a calming influence. One particular study also seemed to show that there were no differences in the levels of activity, social interactions, or mood in children given either artificial sweeteners or sugar; as well as showing that sugar made the children less active.

Sensitivity to sugar
A study published in the *New England Journal of Medicine* in 1994 looked at the effects of diets high in sucrose or aspartame on the behavior and cognitive performance of children aged between six and ten. Apparently these children were recruited for study on the basis that their parents believed their children reacted in a negative way when given sucrose. The researchers found no differences in the behavior of the children when they ate higher-than-normal amounts of sucrose, compared to when they ate diets low in sucrose.

Conclusion
Sugar clearly does give children a rapid supply of energy but that does not mean sugar will make a child hyperactive. The advice of Mark Widome, MD at the American Academy of Pediatrics, is that if you are worried that sugar is causing your child to be out of control rather than just energetic, simply reduce the amount they eat. Whether or not the link between hyperactivity and sugar is justified, it's a great idea to cut down on the amount of sugary foods you or your child eats. These refined carbs are all but empty calories filling you up and leaving no room for you to enjoy more nutritional foods.

Instead of candies, why not share a healthier snack with the child? You can try something like a whole-wheat sandwich filled with either turkey and salad or reduced-fat peanut butter and banana. Or, if you prefer, snack on raw vegetables with a bean dip, or a baked potato with beans, or even French toast made with wholegrain bread (sprinkle with cinnamon instead of syrup).

are all sugars equal?

Fruits and fruit juices

Fresh fruit is not associated with caries because the sugars are held in the cells of the fruit, and are not released until chewing breaks down the cells.

However, the acidity of some fruits and fruit juices (for example, oranges, lemons, and limes) can cause dental erosion. Dental erosion is not the same as dental caries. Erosion is the progressive loss of enamel from the surface of the tooth.

In a fruit juice, the sugars are no longer held within the cells of the fruit. Drinking fruit juice is therefore associated with the development of dental caries especially if the juice is in contact with the teeth for a long period of time, for example, if fed in a baby's bottle or swished around in the mouth.

Another factor that affects the risk of developing caries is the stickiness of the food. Foods like raisins, caramel, or toffees stick to the teeth and so reduce the pH (which means that acid levels increase) in the mouth for a longer period of time. So, it is important that teeth are brushed regularly each day, preferably with fluoride toothpaste, to remove any food sticking to the teeth. Regular brushing and the use of dental floss also removes the plaque coating that collects on the surface of the tooth.

Sugars from milk

Some foods may actually protect our teeth against caries. Milk and, especially, cheese appear to be able to raise pH values in the mouth and so reduce tooth exposure to acid. Milk and cheese are both rich in calcium and phosphate and encourage remineralization through the calcium and phosphate in the mouth when these foods are eaten. They also increase saliva production, which in turn increases the pH level in the mouth. Foods high in fiber may also help to increase the flow of saliva and sugar free chewing gum also stimulates saliva production, and helps to clean the surface of the tooth.

An easy mistake

Imagine a young girl who likes to keep trim by avoiding candy and cookies. Her friends tell her that fruits and vegetables also contain sugars and therefore must also be bad for her. True or false?

Fruits and some vegetables taste sweet and many people think that they must also

Empty Calories

Many people think that molasses are "healthier" than white sugar. Molasses do contain around 1mg of iron per tablespoon (an important mineral for keeping our blood healthy). However, if you were to rely on molasses to meet your daily requirement of 18 mg of iron, then you would need to eat 18 tablespoons of molasses; that's an additional 990 calories!

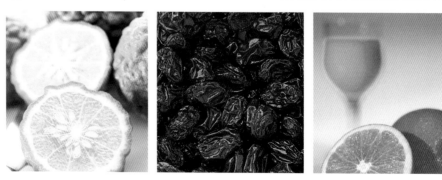

Food	Sugar
1/2 cup canned corn	3 tsp. sugar
12 oz. soda	8 tsp. sugar
1 tbsp. catsup	1 tsp. sugar
8 oz. sweetened yogurt	7 tsp. sugar
2 oz. chocolate	8 tsp. sugar
31/2 oz. ice cream	31/2 tsp. sugar
4 oz. piece of applesauce cake	51/2 tsp. sugar
4 oz. hard candy	20 tsp. sugar
1 tbsp. strawberry jelly	4 tsp. sugar
1/2 oz. unfrosted brownie	3 tsp. sugar
1/2 cup peaches/apricots canned in syrup	31/2 tsp. sugar
1 oz. sugar frosted flakes	2 tsp. sugar
10 oz. bottle root beer	41/2 tsp. sugar
12 oz bottle ginger ale	10 tsp. sugar

contain the same sugars as candy or sodas. While it is true that fruits and vegetables do contain sugars they are, however, packaged with fiber, diluted with plenty of water, and also contain many vitamins, minerals, and healthful phytochemicals and are therefore nutrient dense. They are also "harder to eat" in two ways: that is, they sometimes demand preparation and when eaten the sugar is harder for the body to "get at" immediately. Both "difficulties" tend to reduce calorie intake.

Refined sugars from candy, refined sugar, and syrup, do not contain any fiber and most do not contain any vitamins, minerals, or phytochemicals and so provide nothing but empty calories.

Sugar Substitutes

These include sorbitol, saccharin, and aspartame. They do not provide substantial amounts of calories; these may be good diet buddies if you are watching your calories. A word of warning though, foods that use sugar substitutes may not always be lower in calories than those which use sugars as ingredients. Check your labels carefully.

tips on how to cut down on sugar

- Do not buy fruit canned in light or heavy syrup, always choose those canned in natural juice or water.
- Instead of adding sugar, add flavor to fruit puddings with sweet spices such as cinnamon, nutmeg, allspice, ginger, or clove.
- Gradually reduce the amount of sugar you add to your cereals and coffee—you won't even notice the difference after a few days.
- Reduce the amount of sugars you add to your marinade or cooking by a third or more but do it gradually over the next few weeks.
- Read labels carefully, look out for low-sugar, reduced-sugar, or sugar-free foods. They can help you reduce the overall sugar content of your diet.
- Choose sugar-free or low-sugar versions of juice concentrates and sodas.
- Cut down on the number of sugared drinks you buy and replace them either with water, fruit juice, or diet sodas (as above).
- Choose fresh fruit or reduced-fat popcorn as snacks instead of candy or sweet desserts.

Complex Carbs & Heart Disease

A study published in 1993 followed a large group of women over 10 years and established that an increase in the consumption of wholegrains was linked with a decreased risk of coronary heart disease. In 2002, research published on over 42,000 men, over a period of 12 years, found that a diet rich in wholegrains was associated with a reduced risk of Type II or middle-aged onset diabetes.

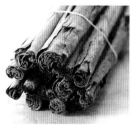
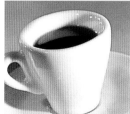

the truth about sugar: questions and answers

1. To avoid sugar, you should drink water instead of soda. True or false?

Answer: True—most of the time, although some bottled waters do contain added sugars. Make sure you check the label and drink calorie-free bottled water or better still tap water—it's free!

2. You should not eat fruit because it contains sugar. True or False?

Answer: False. The sugar contained in fruit is natural, encased in fiber, and diluted with water. Therefore it is a great way to indulge your sweet taste buds while cutting back on added sugar found in processed foods. The fiber provided by fruits also helps to fill you up and curb your mid-morning/mid-afternoon cravings for fatty and sugary snacks.

3. Sugar can revive flagging energy levels. True or false?

Answer: True. Sugary foods, such as chocolate, candy, or cookies, all provide a quick sugar boost but you have to be careful as sugar eaten on its own without other nutrients or fiber will cause glucose levels in your blood to increase rapidly. When they drop back again a few hours later, you may feel like you are in a slump, which in turn can make you crave more food.

3. A healthy diet should not contain any sugar. True or False?

Answer: False. Sugar can be part of a healthy diet. Do not beat yourself up if you have a piece of candy or a cookie occasionally, acknowledge you are going to eat it without feeling guilty and then stop before your next piece.

Mini Quiz: Complex Carbs Or Just Too Complex?

1. At an Italian restaurant, which sauce do you think contains the most amount of complex carbs?

a) pomodoro
b) pesto
c) carbonara

2. Which of the following entrées provides the most fiber?

a) burger and fries
b) beef and bean burrito
c) steak and baked potato

3. Which salad entrée is lower in fat and contains more fiber?

a) Cobb salad with blue cheese dressing
b) Caesar salad
c) Waldorf salad

4. Which sandwich has the most amount of fiber?

a) turkey and salad on rye
b) roast beef and horseradish on crust French
c) ham and cheese on sourdough

Answers
1a, 2b, 3b, 4a

Carbs and sports

Carbs and sports

Carbs are the primary source of fuel for our body, so it should make sense that if we exercise daily we should eat a diet that contains at least a moderate amounts of carbs.

According to the American Dietetic Association, people who exercise on a regular basis should follow a diet that contains a relatively high percentage of energy from carbs and a relatively low percentage of energy from fats. This is because carbs are especially important for endurance exercise. You may remember from Chapter 1 that our glycogen stores in the liver and muscle cells are limited and provide fuel only for a short period of time. As we exercise, these stores are used up, therefore we get tired and exhausted and cannot perform at our best. If our glycogen stores are depleted even before we begin exercising, then tiredness and fatigue will set in rapidly.

So, to get the most out of your hard work when you are training, you should make sure that your pre-exercise glycogen stores are high. Sports nutritionists and exercise physiologists recommend at least 2g of carbs per pound of body weight per day, more for those of you who train a couple of hours a day—around 2.25–3g per pound per day.

where should these carbs come from?

In order to understand what kind of carbs we need when exercising we have to look at the GI again and another concept called "glycemic loading." When concerned with sports performance, important factors to consider are how rapidly glucose is absorbed into the bloodstream (to fuel our muscles and refuel glycogen stores) and the total amount of carbs we eat.

After we consume a high GI food, glucose levels rise quickly in the blood, as a result large amounts of insulin is produced, pushing excess glucose into fat stores. If we eat a large or moderate amount of high GI foods, this will produce a large rise in both blood sugar and insulin (referred to as a "high glycemic load"). Eating a small amount of any carb or a smaller amount of low GI foods will produce a low glycemic load and a more steady and sustained level of blood glucose.

This sustained level of blood glucose is best achieved by eating carbs combined with protein, as this will result in a steady rise in insulin levels, which in turn makes it less likely to promote fat storage. This means that you can eat high GI foods for specific purposes, for example, those athletes who need a quick source of energy before training or diabetics who experience hypoglycemia. In fact, some athletes eat foods such as chips or French fries, in order to fill up their carb reserves before endurance events. Of course, healthier carbs like pasta, potatoes, noodles, rice, fruit, breads, etc. are much more sensible choices as they are lower in fat.

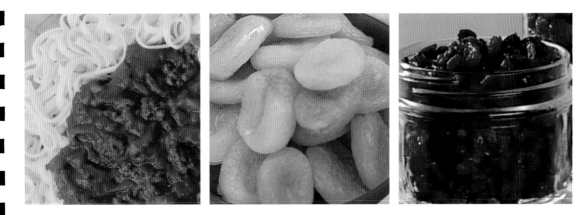

Typical day's menu providing around 2,500 calories	Typical day's menu for an ovo lacto vegetarian providing around 2,500 calories

Breakfast: 1/2 cup granola, 2 tbsp. low-fat yogurt, scant 1 cup low-fat milk, 2/3 cup fruit juice

Breakfast: 2/3 cup fruit juice, 2 slices wholegrain toast, 2 tsp. reduced fat spread, 2 scrambled eggs

Mid morning snack: 1 banana, 1/2 cup strawberries

Mid morning snack: 1 cereal bar

Lunch: 8 1/2 oz. (large) baked potato, 4oz. canned tuna (in brine), 1 cup salad leaves, 1 tbsp. vinaigrette dressing, 1 orange

Lunch: Pasta salad (made with 3 1/2 oz. uncooked pasta), 2 tbsp. kidney beans, 4oz. chopped peppers, 1 tbsp. vinaigrette, 1 orange

Afternoon snack: 1 cereal bar

Afternoon snack: 1 banana, 4oz. berries

Dinner: 7oz. broiled cod, 12oz. sweet potato, 1/2 cup boiled peas, 1/2 cup boiled carrots

Dinner: 4oz. beanburger, 12oz. sweet potato, 1/2 cup boiled carrots, 1/2 cup cooked zucchini

Evening snack: 1/2 mango

Evening snack: 1 pear

During workout: generous 2 cups fruit juice and generous 2 cups water

During workout: generous 2 cups fruit juice and generous 2 cups water

After workout snack: 4 rice cakes, 6 oz. low-fat fruit yogurt

After workout: 1 serving meal replacement product

(Adapted from Bean, A (2003) The Complete Guide to Sports Nutrition, A & C Black, London)

Pre-exercise carbs

The best advice is to choose low GI foods before you exercise and top up with high GI foods during exercise if you train for more than an hour. Low GI meals can be eaten between 2–4 hours before you exercise. Here are some suggestions:

- Bagel or wrap filled with tuna and salad or provolone cheese and salad
- Spaghetti with tomato sauce, vegetables, and meatballs
- Noodles with vegetables and tofu
- Wholegrain cereal with milk

Good carb snacks before exercise include:

- Low-fat yogurt
- Oatmeal and raisin cookie

55

- Dried fruit such as raisins, apricots, etc.
- Fruit smoothie
- Diluted fruit juice

During exercise

Sports nutritionists all agree that it is important to start eating carbs before you feel tired, since it can take at least 30 minutes for glucose to be absorbed into the blood. The American College of Sports Medicine recommends drinking around 5–12fl. oz. ($2/3$–$1^1/2$ cups) of fluid every 15–20 minutes. Carbs that have a high or moderate GI count are ideal. Water is also important; some researchers recommend at least 4 cups of water an hour. Good carb choices while exercising include:

- Isotonic sports drink
- Glucose polymer drink
- Energy/cereal/breakfast bar
- Banana
- Diluted fruit juice (1 part fruit juice diluted with 1 part water)

After exercise

Sports nutritionists recommend refueling as soon as possible after exercise, many suggest eating the equivalent of 0.5g of carbohydrate per pound of body weight during the two hours after exercise. However, for a more efficient refueling of your glycogen stores, exercise physiologists recommend eating at least 50g of carbohydrates every two hours until your next meal. Good carb choices include:

- Fruit smoothie or milkshake
- Sport bar containing both carbs and protein
- Fresh fruit and a glass of milk
- Wholegrain cereal with milk
- Sandwich with salad and chicken or egg
- Yogurt or yogurt drink
- Baked potato with baked beans
- Banana
- Sandwich, pita, bagel, wrap) with tuna or cottage cheese or chicken
- Rice cakes with cottage cheese

What About Coffee And Tea?

Many of us actively avoid drinking coffee and tea because they contain caffeine and caffeine is thought to be a diuretic, with excessive consumption leading to dehydration. However, this was contradicted in an article, published in 2002 in the *International Journal of Sport Nutrition and Exercise Metabolism*, by Professor Lawrence Armstrong, who is a researcher in exercise and environmental physiology. He concluded that moderate caffeine consumption (the equivalent of 1–4 cups of coffee) causes mild diuresis similar to that caused by water. (Diuresis occurs if you drink large volumes of water, which results in an increase of your urine output.) His view is supported by Dr. Heinz Valtin who published a review of scientific literature in the *American Journal of Physiology* in 2002 in which he cites a study that found that caffeinated beverages can be counted toward the daily fluid total.

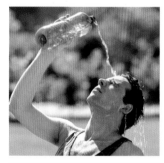
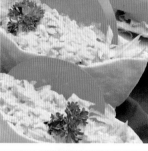
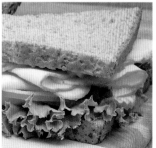
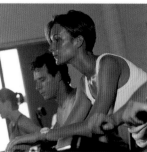

Low carb diets

Low carb diets

a review

According to a poll conducted by Opinion Dynamics Corporation in 2004, around twenty-six million Americans and about 3–4 million in the U.K. follow a strict low-carb diet. Studies in the U.S. have also discovered that more than seventy million people limit their carb intake without actually dieting.

There is no doubt that high-protein, low-carb diets help many people lose weight. In fact. From Bill Clinton or Jennifer Anniston to your neighbor, friend, or partner, most of us are addicted to it, either as passionate proponents or passionate opponents.

The food and drink industry has been quick to respond to this trend and the needs of low-carb dieters, and it has placed over 1,500 new products in our grocery stores. From low-carb beers, burger buns, chips, and breakfast bars to low-carb juice and candy bars. Even restaurants are cashing in and many offer low-carb options.

So, how do these low-carb, high-protein diets work? Some researchers at Harvard claim that those on low-carb, high protein diets actually consume *more* calories but still manage to lose weight. Does this mean that the rules of science been turned upside down? Surely losing weight means eating less and exercising more? Or is it that the combination of high-fat, high-protein foods, produces some sort of magical action in our body, which simply whisks those pounds off but ignores the laws of thermodynamics?

Some plans advocate eating unlimited amounts of meat, fat, dairy, and seafood while avoiding starchy carbs, fruits, and vegetables. Other versions let you include a small amount of carbs and sugars. You will probably have seen people on low-carb, high-protein diets throwing away burger buns and salad leaves and just eating the fatty burgers and mayo. Effectively they are not only eliminating the carbs they are also dumping any nutrients such as fiber, vitamins, or minerals at the same time. How healthy can that really be?

This is the question many health experts around the world are asking. Here is a brief review of a few of the more popular low-carb diets and their (non-) relationships with carbs to provide you with a better idea of what these types of diets are all about.

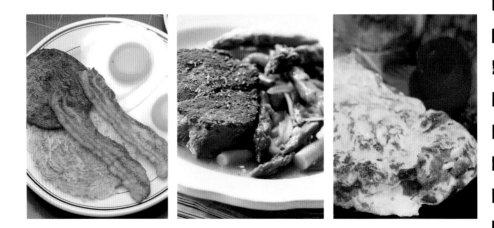

good carbs/bad carbs—the atkins way

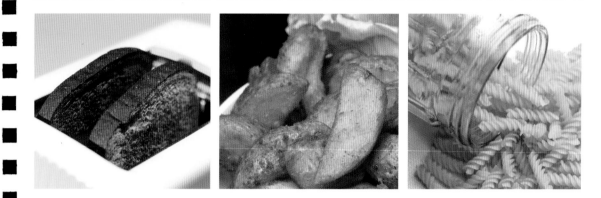

If you have not heard of the Atkins' diet then you have obviously been living on another planet for the last couple of decades. The premise of this diet is that by cutting down on foods high in refined carbohydrates, such as sugar, bread, pasta, cereals, and other low-fat processed foods, you reduce the amount of insulin produced in your body. When there are high levels of insulin in the body, any food you eat is quickly converted and stored as fat, so if you reduce these levels you will lose weight. Those who follow this diet (currently around 40 million people all over the world!) do, in fact, see results in the first few weeks.

Dr. Atkins suggests that most of us eat far too many carbs. He argues that eating high-carb, low-protein, and low-fat meals makes us hungrier and less satisfied than if we ate low-carbohydrate, high-protein, and high-fat foods. This premise is also advocated by government organizations such as the USDA and the British Department of Health, as well as professional bodies such as the American Dietetic Association, American Medical Association, American Heart Association, British Dietetic Association, and British Nutrition Foundation.

So what is the Atkins plan?

The plan focuses on eating foods that are nutrient-dense and unprocessed while augmenting your diet with vitamin and nutrient supplements. It restricts processed and refined carbohydrates and encourages you to eliminate sugar from your diet as this contributes to a slower metabolism. Dr. Atkins' premise is that if you follow his diet and exclude highly refined carbs, you will:

Burn fat first, instead of carbs, and lose weight quickly.
Stave off hunger between meals because high-protein diets are more satiating than high-carb ones. According to his philosophy, as protein is digested slowly in the system, high-protein diets also stabilize blood sugar levels, which can prevent problems such as fatigue, depression, headaches, and joint and muscular pains.
Improve your health because as you burn fat you will also get rid of toxins that are stored in fat cells.

The plan is divided into four distinct stages that promote different rates of weightloss and dietary plans:

- The fortnight induction
- The ongoing weight loss
- Pre-maintenance
- Lifetime maintenance

During the induction phase, carbohydrate consumption is limited to 20g a day; carbs should come mainly from salads and non-starchy vegetables. Once on the weight loss phase you are allowed to increase the amount of carbs you consume through "nutrient-dense" and "fiber-rich" foods by 20g a day in the first week and then 30g a day in the next week until you gradually lose weight. You then subtract 5g of carbohydrate from your daily amount so that you can continue with your sustained weight loss.

The pre-maintenance phase lets you make the transition from losing weight to maintaining your weight by allowing you to increase the amount of carbs you eat every day by 10g increments each week. In the last phase, referred to as lifetime maintenance, the plan allows you to choose from a wider variety of foods but you must still control your carb intake to make sure you maintain your weight.

Typical day's menu for 45g net carbs on the Atkins diet plan

Breakfast: Two slices low-carb French toast with sugar-free pancake syrup, two slices Canadian bacon, 1/2 an orange

Lunch: Tomato stuffed with shrimp salad and chickpea, and vegetable salad

Dinner: Braised short ribs with horseradish sauce, 1/2 cup mashed cauliflower, small green salad with vinaigrette, 1/2 cup raspberries

Snack: 2 oz. almonds

Typical day's menu for 80g net carbs on the Atkins diet plan

Breakfast: Morning muffin with cream cheese and no added sugar/jello, 1/2 cup strawberries

Lunch: Tuna salad, two slices wholegrain bread, small green salad with dressing

Dinner: Lamb chops with tomatoes and olives, brown rice pilaf, one chocolate chip and oatmeal cookie

Snack: Celery stuffed with 1 tbsp. sugar-free peanut butter

Typical day's menu for 60g net carbs on the Atkins diet plan

Breakfast: 1 cup plain yogurt, 2 tbsp. wheatgerm, 1/2 cup strawberries

Lunch: Salmon salad with arugula on one slice of wholegrain bread

Dinner: Chile Blanco (means white chile containing no tomatoes), low-carb tortilla, 1/2 cup watermelon

Snack: 1/2 oz. hard cheese

Typical day's menu for 100g net carbs on the Atkins diet plan

Breakfast: 2 slices light rye toast, 1/2 cup plain whole yogurt, 1/2 cup blueberries

Lunch: Large green salad with 1/2 cup beans

Dinner: Broiled steak, 1/3 cup whole-wheat pasta, pineapple-mango layer cake

Snack: 1 kiwi fruit

Source: Men plans from Dr. Robert C. Atkins (2003) Atkins for Life: The next level: permanent weight loss and good health. Pan books

How the diet works

How the Atkins diet helps you to lose weight is simple. According to its creator, when you eat very few carbohydrates (which are commonly your main source of energy), the body goes into what is called a "ketogenic state" where it must rely on stored fat for energy. As a result, you burn fat quickly and begin to lose weight. This process also makes the body produce compounds called ketones (which are not considered to be dangerous) that initially give dieters a what many describe as a "buzz" or euphoric feeling; and bad breath! According to most Atkins followers they do not feel deprived on low-carb diets for the first several days because they are eating meals high in fat. Some people may get withdrawal symptoms because, according to Atkins' theory, they are "addicted" to sugar, wheat, and caffeine.

These withdrawal symptoms often include fatigue, feeling faint, palpitations, cold sweats, and headaches. Atkins claims these symptoms usually disappear within three days and he advises that you ride through them. Many who have tried the Atkins diet say it helped them lose weight much more quickly than conventional low-fat diets.

Critics of the diet

Health experts say that the real reason low-carb diets actually lead to quick weight loss is because dieters have to restrict many of the foods they eat, including fruits, vegetables, breads, and cereals. They also say that it is difficult to maintain this kind of diet over a long period of time precisely because your choice of foods is limited.

In a recent scientific review on popular diets, published in *Obesity Research* in 2000, the lead researchers doctors, Freedman, King, and Kennedy, concluded that during the induction phase of the diet, most of the rapid weight loss is due to the loss of water rather than fat. As fat is broken down instead of glycogen the body's metabolic rate can decrease by up to 20 percent after six weeks, so after a while your body becomes less efficient at burning off fat.

The researchers also concluded that the diet is deficient in fiber, vitamin E, iron, magnesium, and folate, and excessive in total fat, saturated fat, cholesterol, vitamin A, phosphorous, and potassium. Additionally, they reported that the Atkins diet contains only around 25 percent of the recommended daily intake of fiber, but supplies 55–65 percent fat, compared to a 35 percent fat intake currently recommended by both the American and British governments. Critically, high-fat and low-fiber intakes have been identified as risk factors for cancers of the colon, breast, and stomach.

In the *American Journal of Dietetics* in 2004, Dean Ornish, Clinical professor of Medicine at the University of California and president of the Preventive Medicine Research Institute, wrote a commentary entitled *Was Atkins Right?*

According to Ornish, both he and Dr. Atkins agreed that many people eat too many simple carbs. But while Ornish advocates substituting simple carbs with complex (unrefined) ones, Atkins prescribes replacements for these carbs with high-fat, high-protein foods such as bacon, sausage, pork rinds, and brie.

Proponents of the diet

Those people who do support the Atkins philosophy say that critics are wrong when they assert that the plan never allows you to eat carbs and is just a diet of red meat and saturated fats.

According to Dr. Stuart Trager, medical director of Atkins Nutritionals, "Atkins For Life shatters the myth that a low-carb regime is a red meat diet. With more

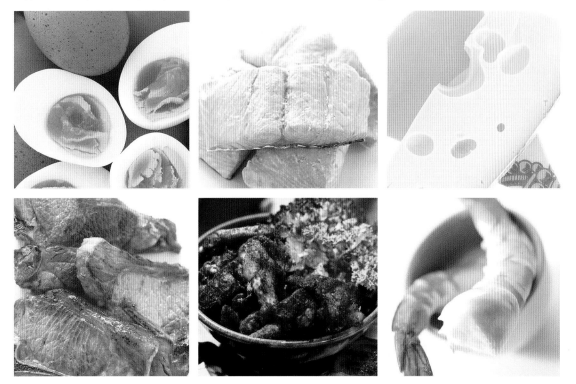

than 125 recipes and six months of menu plans, the Atkins Nutritional Approach features pork, chicken, fish, and vegetarian dishes, as well as those for beef and other red meats. Anyone who limits their diet to bun-less bacon cheeseburgers and inch-thick steaks is not doing Atkins correctly." He suggests following ten simple rules:

- Count your daily Net Carbs (total carbs minus fiber).
- Stay at or below your Atkins Carbohydrate Equilibrium (ACE). This is the amount of carbs you can eat a day while neither gaining nor losing pounds.
- Adjust your ACE as needed.
- Eat primarily whole, unprocessed foods.
- Stay away from added sugar, bleached white flour, hydrogenated oils, and any types of junk food.
- Do not go for more than 4–6 waking hours without a meal or snack.
- Exercise regularly.
- Take a multivitamin and mineral supplements, and essential fatty acids.
- Drink a minimum of eight 7fl. oz. (scant 1 cup) of glasses of water every day.
- Never let yourself gain more than 5lb.

Scientific studies showing the benefits of the Atkins diet plan have shown that the diet helped a group of people lose an average of 21 lb., lower their cholesterol and triglyceride levels, and raise HDL ("good" cholesterol) over a period of four months. Advocates of the diet say that people at high risk of chronic disease such as cardiovascular disease, hypertension, and diabetes will actually see a marked improvement. Several studies have also shown that men and women lost twice the weight on the Atkins plan, compared to conventional low-fat diets.

good carbs/bad carbs—the south beach way

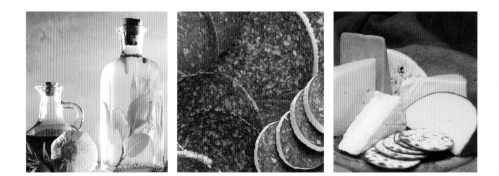

The South Beach plan is based on the principle that certain types of carbohydrates cause people to gain weight. Carbohydrates are allowed on the diet but are divided into good and bad categories. As a general guideline, all refined foods, like cookies and pasta, are classed as the "bad."

Dr. Agatston, the creator of this diet, proposes that bad carbs make you feel temporarily full by causing your blood sugar levels to rise rapidly. When levels start to decline, you then start to feel lethargic and hungry again. These bad carbs are also classed as foods with a high glycemic index (refer back to Chapter 4 for details on the GI).

The good and bad dichotomy extends to fats, with monounsaturated fats (like those from olive and rapeseed oils) which are classed as good fats and saturated fats (such as fatty meats and dairy products) as the bad.

What does this mean?
The South Beach Diet claims that it is not low in carbs or low in fat, but that weight loss is

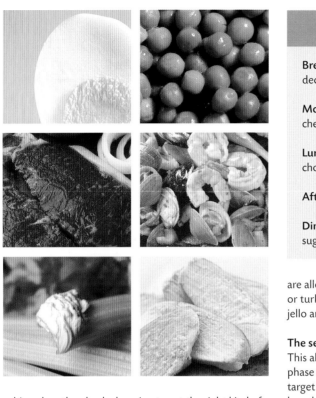

Typical day's menu on Phase I of South Beach diet

Breakfast: Two poached eggs with lean bacon and decaffeinated tea or coffee

Morning snack: Celery with 3 oz. low-fat cottage cheese

Lunch: Red bell pepper stuffed with feta and chopped vegetables

Afternoon snack: A small wedge of low-fat cheese

Dinner: Poached salmon with Greek salad and sugar-free jello with low-fat topping

achieved on the plan by learning to eat the right kind of carbs and the right fat. The plan advocates a life-long regime to help you to learn to live without the bad carbs and fat. The diet does not require you to measure what you eat in ounces, calories, or anything else. What the guidelines do dictate is that your meals should be of a normal size, that is, large enough to satisfy your hunger but no more than that. The diet is divided into three phases as follows:

The first phase
This is aimed at banishing your cravings for the bad carbs and fat. It lasts for two weeks and is based on a restricted plan of three meals and two snacks a day. This phase promises a weight loss of between 8–13lb.

What's out: Bread, potatoes, pasta, rice, or baked products. Fruit, fruit juices, milk, yogurt, full-fat cheese, butter, alcohol, candies, cakes, and any sugary foods.

What's in: Lean cuts of meat, poultry, fish, shellfish, eggs, low-fat or fat-free cheese, and some nuts. Low glycaemic index vegetables (for example, broccoli, cabbage, cucumber, celery), olive or rapeseed oil. For snacks you

are allowed to have low-fat cheese with celery, cucumber, or turkey slices, and for desserts, you can have sugar-free jello and dishes made with low-fat ricotta cheese.

The second phase
This allows you to reintroduce carbs into your diet. This phase should be followed until you have reached your target weight. Again, your dietary plan at this stage is based on having three meals a day with two snacks and a dessert for dinner.

Back in: Fruits except bananas, pineapple, raisins, and watermelon. Limited amounts of wholegrain bread, wholegrain cereals such as brown rice, whole-wheat pasta, low-fat dairy products, wine, and limited amounts of bittersweet or semisweet chocolate.

What's out: Refined breads and cereals, white potatoes, beets, carrots, and corn kernels.

Your weight loss should slow down during this stage in comparison to phase one. You are given the option to

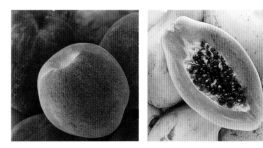

Typical day's menu on Phase II of South Beach diet

Breakfast: $1/2$ grapefruit and 1 slice whole-wheat toast topped with low-fat cheese and decaffeinated coffee or tea

Morning snack: $3^1/2$oz. low-fat yogurt

Lunch: Greek salad with whole-wheat pita

Afternoon snack: 1 apple

Dinner: Stir-fried chicken with vegetables and mixed salad and strawberries with low-fat cream

Source: Men plans from Arthur Agatson (2003) The South Beach Diet: A doctor's plan for fast and lasting weight loss. Headline

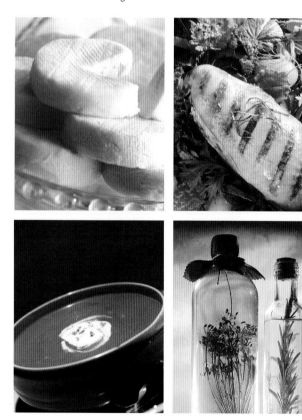

continue phase one for another week if you think you can maintain the strictness of it. But, you are advised to transfer to phase three so that you don't get bored and revert to your bad eating habits.

The third phase

By this stage you should be at your ideal weight. The third phase is not aimed at promoting weight loss but adapting the diet to become part of a healthy ongoing lifestyle regimen. This phase does allow for more variety but it is basically more of the same from the previous two phases. You are allowed to fall off the wagon occasionally and go back to phase one if you feel it is necessary and then go back to phase three.

Restaurant strategies

Dr. Agatston devotes an entire chapter of his book on how to eat in a restaurant. During the first phase of the diet, it would probably be quite difficult to eat out, although it's possible. For example, you can limit yourself to a plain broiled chicken breast and a leafy salad with olive oil dressing. While on the first phase of the diet the temptation to eat breads, deep fried foods, and other banned items may be too great unless you have steel willpower. Dining out during the second and third phase will be easier, since you are allowed to have alcohol then too.

When you do eat out, Dr. Agatston proposes that you eat a protein snack such as low-fat cheese fifteen minutes before you are due to arrive at the restaurant. This starts the process of filling you up so that by the time the waiter arrives, you will not want to order the entire menu.

Some other useful tips include drinking soup or consommé as soon as you arrive. This does the same thing as the protein snack, since it takes about twenty minutes or so before signals from your stomach start channelling through to your brain to tell you that you are full. Of course, according to the rules of the diet, rice and potatoes are off limits at any restaurant as well as no fries or fast food.

Dr. Agatston's patients with diabetes or heart problems who followed the diet lost weight, had lower levels of bad blood cholesterol, and their insulin resistance improved.

Once you understand what foods to mix and which ones to avoid, you can create your own version of the plan, so that you enjoy the foods you eat and stay on the diet. There is emphasis on adopting an exercise regime, which will improve blood pressure, blood cholesterol, and general health. Overall, this plan is good for people who have the willpower to cut out favorites for a while but who don't want to feel like they are on a diet for life.

good carbs/bad carbs—the carbohydrate addicts way

Creators of the Carbohydrate Addicts diet *The Carbohydrate Addict's Lifespan Program*, doctors Richard and Rachael Heller say that because of an addiction to carbohydrates, almost three-quarters of everyone who is overweight finds themselves fighting a losing battle against weight loss. They assert that excessive insulin is the route cause of this addiction, in fact the rise of insulin levels caused by eating certain types of foods actually induces the "carbohydrate addict" to eat more carbs. Their book includes a quiz to help you assess whether you are an addict or not.

The diet

The plan does not allow you to have any carbs at all for either breakfast or lunch. These two meals should consist solely of protein and non-starchy vegetables. You are allowed to have a reward meal once a day for dinner. This meal should consist of $1/3$ protein, $1/3$ carb, and $1/3$ non-starchy vegetables, plus you are allowed to eat desserts. The only snag is that you have to finish eating the meal within one hour. Plus, if you must have seconds or thirds, then you have to serve yourself equal amounts of protein, carbs, and non-starchy vegetables and not just carbs.

The husband and wife team state that once you have been following these rules in the proscribed way for a suitable length of time, your cravings for carbs will disappear. However, if you still have cravings after a week or so, you are asked to check that you are following the rules accurately.

Tips for success

- Watch your portion sizes since they aren't specified. Overeating at any meal or on any diet plan means you're going eat more calories which won't lead to weight loss.
- You should choose lean meats as your protein source and vary them. For example try pulses, legumes, tofu, poultry, fish, and eggs rather than just having meat.

This plan is not recommended by any health or dietary organizations and a critic of the diet, Neal Barnard, MD, President of the Physicians Committee for Responsible Medicine, says: "This diet addresses a problem that is not even remotely the problem for most overweight people ... it would be much more effective to repair the body's ability to handle carbohydrates rather than demonizing them, and this is done by cutting fat out of the diet, boosting fiber, and choosing those carbohydrates such as whole grains and vegetables that release glucose slowly—and, finally, by adding exercise to your routine."

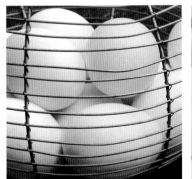
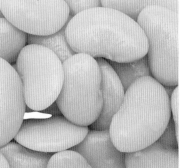
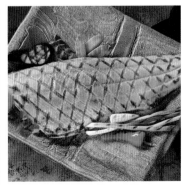

good carbs: bad carbs—the zone way

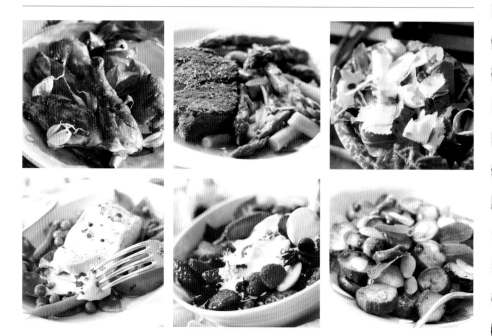

The Zone Diet (or 40-30-30 plan) follows a dietary regime that promotes a 40 percent carbohydrate, 30 percent protein, and 30 percent fat plan. The diet works on the premise that 100,000 years ago, our ancestors were meat eaters and so our bodies were primarily designed to deal with digesting a carnivorous-based diet. As we have evolved, more carbohydrates have been introduced into our diet, thus causing an imbalance in the natural order of things. The creator of the plan, Dr. Barry Spears, says that the reason why we put on weight can be attributed to the grains and starches in our diet such as pasta, rice, breads, and potatoes. The Zone Diet suggests a return to the prehistoric diet where meat, fruits, and vegetables were the main dietary items. So, a no-grains zone!

Dr. Spears says that his plan is "not a diet, but a life long hormonal control strategy." The Zone website (www.zoneperfect.com) states that "the more insulin you produce the fatter you become," and proposes that diets that have a high carb intake lead to obesity. The plan lays the ultimate blame on grains. The premise is that the introduction of grain into the diet has made mankind "shrink" from not having enough protein and that chronic illness such as heart disease, arthritis, and obesity are the result of carbohydrates and insulin.

Typical day's menu on the Zone Diet

Breakfast: Egg and Fruit

Lunch: Grilled/broiled Chicken Salad

Afternoon Snack: 1/2 a ZonePerfect Bar

Dinner: Baked Fish and Vegetables

Evening Snack: 1/2 a ZonePerfect Bar

Source: www.zone.com

How does the Zone Diet Work?
The Zone Diet works by calculating the correct ratio of carbohydrates to proteins and fats in

order to control the amount of insulin circulating in the blood. Too much insulin increases fat storage and inflammation in the body (which can cause obesity, type-II diabetes, and heart disease). Through the regulation of blood sugar, your body is allowed to burn off excess fat.

The plan recommends that you avoid of high-fat foods and carbohydrates such as grains, starches, and pastas. Fruits and vegetables are the preferred source of carbs and monounsaturated fats, such as that from olive oil, almonds, and avocados, should be your ideal choice of fats. The central tenet to this diet plan is the presence of compounds called eicosanoids. Eicosanoids include prostaglandins, thromboxanes, and leukotrienes, which have various physiological effects in the body. Dr. Sears theory suggests that there are both "good" and "bad" eicosanoids, and that following the Zone Diet will change the ratio of good eicosanoids to bad.

Critics of the Zone Diet
Many health experts, including those from the American Heart Association (AHA), say that the Zone Diet has not been proven to be effective in the long term for weight loss. They also state that it is complicated to follow; that by eliminating certain foods from your diet it means that your need for certain essential vitamins and minerals will not be met; that it is expensive and time consuming to follow. The AHA is also concerned that the ratio of protein is too high even though the fat ratio is low.

Advocates of the Zone Diet
Advocates for the Zone Diet include high profile celebrities like Madonna, Jennifer Aniston, and Minnie Driver. Some health experts say that the Zone's recommendations do not stray far from the USDA's dietary guidelines.

good carbs: bad carbs—the sugar busters way

This diet was first published in 1995. The authors cite sugar and insulin as the culprits that are preventing us from losing weight even though we follow strict diets and exercise.

The authors propose that it is sugar and not fat that is the cause of our excess baggage. Furthermore, refined sugars are stated to be "toxic" to the body because they spike insulin levels, which can lead to insulin resistance, high blood sugar levels, increased cravings for sugary foods, and increased production of cholesterol in the liver. The authors also state that high GI foods contribute toward our bodies developing insulin resistance and that restricting calories does not necessarily lead to weight loss.

What is the Sugar Busters diet plan?
The Sugar Busters! Cut Sugar to trim fat diet by Leighton H. Steward, Morrison C. Bethea, Sam S. Andrews, and Luis A. Balart is based on a plan that follows containing 30 percent protein, 40 percent fat, and 30 percent carbohydrates diet. It recommends that you eat according to the Glycemic Index if you want to achieve weight loss.

What's in: Lean red meat such as. beef, pork, poultry, fish, wild game, olive oil, dairy foods, nuts, non-starchy vegetables (but not carrots), most fruits (but not bananas), low or reduced fat dairy products without

added sugar. Small amounts of wholegrain bread, whole-wheat pasta, and oats, wholegrains, chocolate, nuts, and artificial sweeteners.

Typical day's menu on the Sugar Busters diet
Breakfast: Orange or $1/2$ a grapefruit, hot oatmeal, coffee, or tea
Lunch: Turkey and Swiss cheese on rye, wholegrain, or pumpernickel bread with mustard and/or thinly spread light mayonnaise, lettuce, and tomato, diet drink, tea, or water
Afternoon snack: 12 grapes
Dinner: Ground beef cooked in no-added-sugar tomato sauce with whole-wheat pasta and Romano or Parmesan cheese, steamed spaghetti, squash and/or zucchini, romaine lettuce salad, and water
Dessert: Sugar-free yogurt or ice cream

Source: www.sugarbusters.com

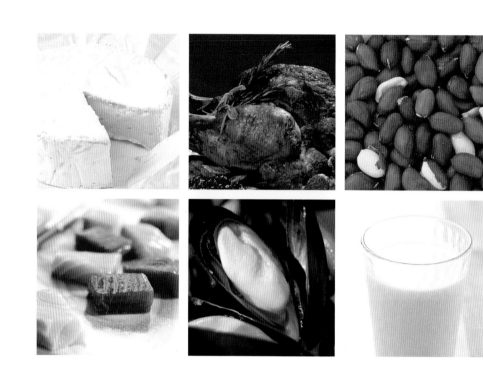

What's out: Potatoes, white bread, white pasta, white rice, all refined sugar, banana, carrots, corn, popcorn, and beets.

Critics of the diet:

According to North Western University in the U.S., the Sugar Busters diet plan has several nutritional shortcomings. The university states that the diet:

• Is low in essential nutrients including vitamin D, vitamin E, calcium, and iron.

• Eliminates a wide range of foods which contain carbohydrates, including some fruits. They feel that long-term compliance to avoiding fruits, baked goods, and candy is difficult for many people.
• Offers many protein sources which are high in dietary cholesterol and saturated fat.
• Lacks phytochemicals derived from carbohydrate-rich plant foods.
• Is difficult to follow long-term for those who enjoy eating candy, breads, fruits, or other carbohydrate-containing foods.

beware the quick fix

It's thought that more than 54 million Americans are currently on a diet. Although some manage to lose weight, only a small percentage—around five percent—succeed in keeping the weight off over a long period of time. Miserable statistics!

No wonder most of us are continuously searching for a fast and easy fix. But take a minute to stop and think what effects quick-fix diets might have on your future health.

Being more active in daily life helps to lift mood and self-esteem, regulate (not increase) appetite, maintain muscle, and make long-term success more likely. Some quick-fix diets are short-term. Other diets are too rigid to sustain for long. They may also be nutritionally inadequate and could lead to problems such as iron-deficiency or poor bone health.

Imagine if your vacuum hose was

broken, a quick fix would just be to tape it over and hope for the best until it breaks again the next time. A longer-term solution would obviously be to replace it with a new hose.

While I am not suggesting you replace your body with newer parts, far from it, what I am suggesting is that you take some time and think about adopting a long-term, realistic, and healthy solution, rather than opting for a magic solution.

The International Food Information Council, (based in Washington, DC) say that you can spot a fad diet because they usually:

Claim, or imply, that you will achieve a large or quick weight loss of more than 1 or 2 lb. per week. Slow, gradual weight loss increases the chance of success and of keeping weight off over the long term.
Promote magical or miracle foods. No foods can undo the long-term effects of overeating and not exercising, neither can they magically melt away fat.
Restrict or eliminate certain foods, recommend certain foods in large quantities, insist on eating specific food combinations, or offer rigid, inflexible menus.

Suggest that weight can be lost and maintained without exercise and other lifestyle changes.
Rely heavily on undocumented case histories, testimonials, and anecdotes but have no scientific research to back claims.
Contradict what most trusted health professional groups say, or make promises that sound too good to be true.

Conclusion

You should always consult with your doctor or dietician before undertaking any dietary plan, and high-protein, low-carb diets should be followed under medical supervision. Remember that in order to achieve successful weight loss you will also need to increase your levels of physical activity and get as much support from others as possible.

Studies have shown that dieters typically lost more weight when they linked up with the Internet—there are many websites that act as virtual dieting support communities, for example www.ivillage.com, where dieters can share success or failures, good practices, and tips for success.

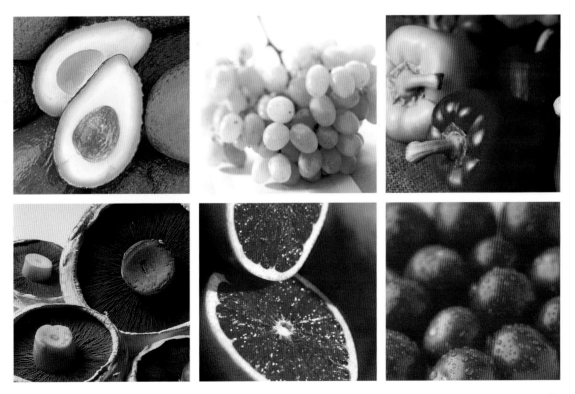

make carbs your best friend

It is much easier than you think to find the right carbs—here are some tips on how to choose the right carbs and enjoy your food.

The diet
Choose a diet that consists mostly of moderate to low GI foods, that is, unrefined wholegrain foods which take the body longer to digest and so will not lead to a rush of glucose into the blood. But don't beat yourself up if you have the occasional low GI food.

Sizing
The only supersizing you will do from now on is to supersize your fruit and vegetable portions.

Eating out
Watch your portion sizes especially when you are eating out. It might help to measure out recommended portions of foods from the different food groups so that you can visualize how much say one cup of vegetables are or how big a 1oz. portion of beans is when ordering your meal.

Cravings
Acknowledge that there will be situations that will trigger your desire to crave and eat sugary, fatty "comfort" foods. Have a mental list of what you can do to distract yourself from bingeing on refined carbs.

Swapping foods
Next time you reach out to put a bag of white rice in your shopping cart, swap it for a pack of brown rice instead.

Food labels
Check the amount of fiber and sugar each food contains, as well as the number of calories if you are watching your weight. This will add more time to your grocery shopping but it is worth the effort—you are investing in your future health and there is nothing more important than that!

Fiber
Leave the peel on fruits and vegetables if you want to gain the maximum amount of fiber from them. If you are worried about pesticides and other chemical contaminants choose organic if your budget allows.

Variety
Eat a wide variety of foods, you will benefit from a more diverse range of nutrients, essential vitamins, minerals, and phytochemicals, which will keep you healthy and your diet interesting.

Enjoy your food
If you really hate the taste of whole-wheat pasta but like eating whole-wheat bread, then so be it. We are not at school now, we do not need to be forced to eat up!

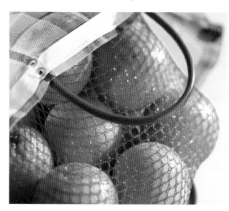

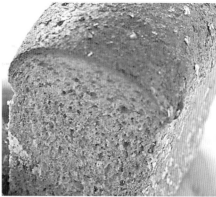

Eating out

Eating out

Temptations all around: How to watch your calories as well as making healthy carb choices when eating out.

It is all too easy to binge on donuts, cookies, and ice cream when you're out and about, and when you need to grab food on the go between school runs and grocery shopping, so it makes sense for you to be prepared for eventualities. There are some simple rules that can help such as always eat a snack before you go grocery shopping, that way you're less tempted to want to buy anything that's on sale. Snack on some rye crispbreads topped with sliced apple and low-fat cottage cheese before you go or if you're short of time, fill a small plastic container with low-fat granola or air popped popcorn to snack on in the car.

what about eating out in restaurants?

Do the following statements sound like you?

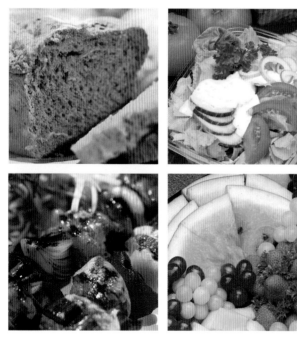

- You want to order everything on the menu—and feel as if you have been deprived if you only have an appetizer and an entrée.

- You smother the bread rolls with butter and eat them all before your appetizer arrives.
- You eye up your partner's or your children's leftovers and then eat it all even though you've eaten all the food on your plate.
- You avoid the salad bar at all costs because you think it's too healthy.
- You will only order deep-fried appetizers and high-fat entrées and then pig out on a high-fat, sugary desserts whatever cuisine you're eating—all without a vegetable or fruit in sight.
- You feel deprived if your meal is smaller than someone else's on your table.

If you answered yes to any of the above then help is at hand with the following restaurant guide. Some establishments are likely to offer some of the following options so ask for them if you don't see them immediately:

lower in fat, for example, reduced calories salad dressings, skim or low-fat milk, baked or broiled food
lower in salt, for example, salt substitutes
higher in fiber, for example, salads, wholegrain breads

lower in sugar, for example, low-calorie sweeteners, fresh fruit, yogurt

heart healthy, for example, low-cholesterol eggs, lean meat, skinless chicken

Here is some general advice that is easy to follow whereever you are eating out:

Try to order only what you need. Sometimes our eyes are bigger than our appetite and we end up finishing meals when we're already full.

Try to eat the same portion as you would at home. This means that you will have to be careful of jumbo, deluxe, supersize, or giant portions, as these mean extra food and therefore extra calories that you don't need.

Try to eat slowly. This will let you enjoy your food more, and it gives your body the opportunity to alert you to when you are full, and it also helps digestion.

Ask for sauces, gravy, and dressings "on the side." This will help you to limit the amount you put on your food

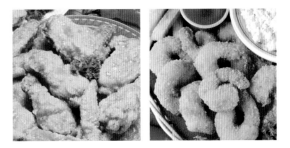

and enables you to control your calorie intake.

Strip breaded or fried foods. These contain a lot of fat, so if you're desperate to have deep fried items, eat one with the coating and then peel off the outer coating of the remaining items.

Pass on the French fries. Ask for a double order of a vegetable instead of French fries or choose something else from the salad bar. When you're at the salad bar, watch out that you do not overload your plate with diet saboteur high-fat items such as bacon bits, cheeses, mayo, and croutons.

specific tips

When eating out in restaurants you are always going to be surrounded by temptation and this can be very miserable when you are trying to watch your wasteline. But dining out doesn't have to be hell and it doesn't mean you can't enjoy your food. You simply have to remind yourself to be aware of what you are ordering, make sensible menu choices, and don't overindulge. Here are some specific tips to help you to enjoy eating out without the guilt:

Italian

Eating Italian is often synonymous with pasta and pizza. Although pasta and pizza dough on their own are low in fat and low in calories, adding pesto, carbonara, other creamy sauces, cheese, pine kernels, etc., means adding extra calories and extra fat. Additionally, pasta and pizza dough are usually made with refined flour which means that they're going to be low in fiber, so if you're going to indulge, choose pasta and pizza as an appetizer rather

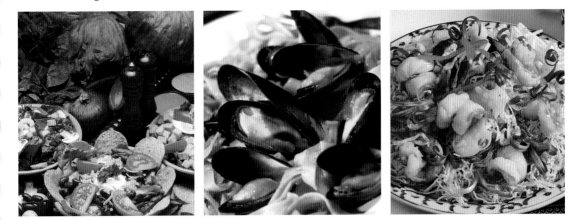

than as an entrée. To bump up your fiber content, serve yourself an extra large portion of salad with low-fat dressing and fill up with a hearty minestrone soup.

Chinese

Chinese is a popular cuisine to choose when eating out, but watch out for the extra large portions of rice and noodles. These are usually loaded with oil, particularly if you order fried rice or fried noodles. If you want to eat these then order a portion and share it with a friend. Soups are always great to fill up on before the entrée's come so order those which have veggies in them, such as hot and sour soup or crab and corn soup. Fresh fruit is usually preferable as desserts rather than candied apples or fortune cookies.

Family Restaurants

There are some great family-style restaurants, which will suit many people's budgets. Portions will be large so stick to two appetizers and choose two entrees if you're a family of four, if there's any left over, don't take it away, as you are likely to eat it in the car before you even get home. Choose whole-wheat pitas or whole-wheat bread and skip the butter and mayo. Remember croissants are high in fat so keep these for very occasional treats. Pile your plate high with salad and choose a low-fat dressing; remember coleslaw and potato salads are off limits as they are loaded with mayo. There is usually some great vegetable soups, such as minestrone, so there's no excuse to choose the creamy calorie dense ones! Vegetable-based burgers may sound like a good higher fiber substitute for a meat burger but be careful as this might be at the expense of extra calories, most are deep-fried so check with your waiter before you order.

Fast food

Fast foods are a way of life for most of us nowadays and many restaurants provide drive-thrus which are accessible, convenient, and cheap. If you are going to eat in one of these restaurants don't be tempted to order high-fat, high-calorie items like Danish or taco shells. Choose a small whole-wheat or multigrain bagel instead. The salad bar is again a great choice provided you steer clear of the high-fat dressings. Baked potatoes shared with a friend are great carb choices over French fries but top these with low-fat yogurt and vegetables rather than with cheese and butter. Similarly, pretzels are a much better alternative to high-fat potato chips.

French food

Nouvelle cuisine used to mean smaller helpings and lighter sauces but the portion sizes seem to be increasing with our super-sizing culture and perception of value for money these days. Soups like consommé, or French onion soup (skip the cheese-topped croutons) make great appetizers, as do mixed green salads with low-fat dressing. If whole-wheat or multigrain bread is available choose these and share with friends but skip the

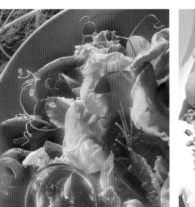
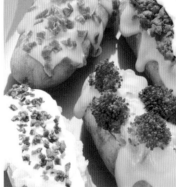
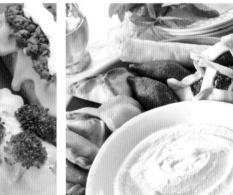

butter. Fruits make great desserts; you don't have to drown them with cream or ice cream to enjoy them.

Greek and middle eastern food

Traditional dishes, such asTzatziki (yogurt and cucumber dip) with whole-wheat pita make a great appetizer to share with friends. Hummus (chickpea dip) in theory is also a great carb choice but it is often drenched with oil and so is not so friendly to those watching their waistlines. Couscous or bulgur wheat with vegetables are fantastic starchy substitutes for white rice but, as always, watch your portion size and ask the chef to hold back on the butter or oil. Phyllo pastry is very tempting, it tastes heavenly, is light and crisp, but contains sugar and an inordinate amount of butter, so steer clear of pies, savory, or sweet pastries. Even though they may seem good carb choices as they're often filled with spinach or fruit.

Indian food

Many indian dishes traditionally contain legumes and vegetables and may sound like an ideal cuisine to have but most are prepared with ghee (clarified butter) which can make certain dishes calorie-dense. Try to choose appetizers such as papadums and raitas (cucumber and yogurt dip with spices). Watch out for vegetable samosas and pakoras (deep-fried vegetables in batter). Although these foods have a good fiber content, they are deep-fried and so are calorie-dense. If you are a family of four choose one protein entrée (meat and preferably tomato-based) and two vegetable entrées (dahls and vegetable curries such as cauliflower with peas and tomatoes) to share. Fresh fruit, especially mango, always provide great alternatives to kulfi (very rich and sweet Indian ice cream) and Indian desserts.

Japanese Food

Japanese portions are usually smaller but that shouldn't give you an excuse to eat more! Although vegetable tempura are higher in fiber than if you choose miso soup, they are also higher in calories. Therefore, if you choose tempura as an appetizer then you should go for something that is low in fat for the entrée, such as soba or buckwheat noodles in soup, topped with something that is low in fat like tofu and vegetables. Sushi, although it is low in fat, tends to be low in fiber so remember not to overindulge and choose a side salad to make up for the lost fiber.

Mexican Food

Nachos, fried taco shells, and tortilla chips are all loaded with fat, so you really need to try and avoid them—corn tortillas are better substitutes. Guacamole, although made with avocados, is also high in fat so remember that if you are watching your weight. If you must have an appetizer a great choice are whole-wheat breadsticks with a salsa dip.

Steakhouses

Salads make great low calorie accompaniments to a small lean steak. Remember to ask for a low-fat dressing on the side. Steamed vegetables are also good, nutritious choices as long as they're not overcooked. Also ask the chef to hold back on the butter. Fruit sherberts or frozen non-fat yogurt make good substitutes for apple pie and ice cream.

Vietnamese and Thai food

Going to eat in either a Thai or Vietnamese restaurant can be a good choice for those watching their carbs or dieting in any way, because dishes are traditionally meant

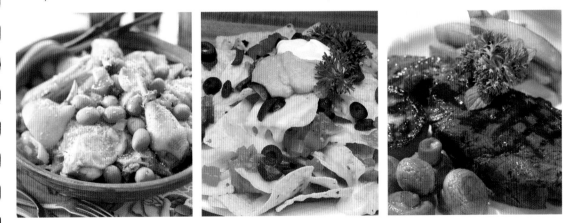

for sharing. This helps you watch your portions for fear of offending your fellow diners!

Deep fried spring rolls, although delicious, are high in fat. Great alternatives to these are fresh spring rolls and this gives you a good opportunity to experiment with new flavors and tastes. Bear in mind the soft translucent spring roll wrappers are made with refined rice flour but if you fill them up with loads of fresh vegetables and tasty herbs, this will make up for the lack of fiber in them. Make these your main entrées rather than appetizers since starchy carb choices, such as sticky rice and rice noodles, don't contain much fiber (though It is often difficult to eat Thai curries without rice).

Most curries traditionally contain high-fat coconut milk or cream and peanuts, so you will be able to watch your calories by limiting these. Hot and sour soups contain vegetables without coconut milk and so are lower in calories and a much better choice.

Finish off your meal with a plate of fresh tropical fruits or fruit ice, rather than coconut ice cream or sweet sticky rice, which are, of course, calorie-dense.

Breakfasts

Eating breakfast is a great start to the day as it revs up your metabolism after a night of fasting. If you don't eat breakfast there is a tendency for you to crave a quick sugar hit by the middle of the morning. (But beware the sheer volume and choice offered in some hotels—make a choice before you get to the dining room.)

Your first choice should be a piece of fresh fruit and fruit juice. You can then alternate each day with either wholegrain cereals (not high-fat granolas) and fat-free milk or multigrain bagels with reduced-fat cream cheese or hot oatmeal, grits, or cream of wheat.

Party food

It is all too easy to pile your plate up high with deep fried appetizers and gorge on low-fiber, high-fat snacks when you are at a social function. Couple this with a glass or 10 of wine and you have succeeded in eating yet another "meal" that will undoubtedly make you feel too full and unhappy with yourself.

A really easy piece of advice to remember is to eat something before you go out. You can, for example, snack on an open sandwich, try something like a slice of pumpernickel bread or multigrain bread topped with cucumber and smoked salmon or papaya and prosciutto ham. When you get to the party, ask for a glass of iced water and alternate this with diluted fruit juice or wine.

It is also a good idea to try and position yourself on the opposite side of the room to the buffet table to so that it is difficult for you to go back to it frequently and the temptation is farther away! This may seem ridiculous but it really can save you eating while distracted. If you do eat at the party don't pile your plate high with food and try to choose vegetable crudités with low-fat dips and limit yourself to only one deep fried processed snack.

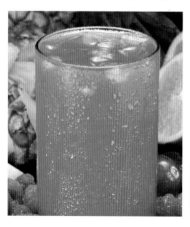
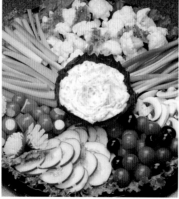
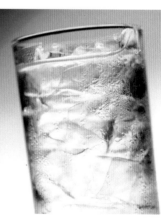

Special diets

Special diets

Advice and tips for specific dietary needs.

From the earlier chapters you will now understand what carbs are, what foods contain which carbs, and how these are normally digested and dealt with by the body. There are, however, certain physical conditions that may prevent some of us from dealing with carbs in the "normal" way, such as diabetes, lactose intolerance, and hypoglycemia. Other conditions where carbs are important include pre-menstrual syndrome (PMS), polycystic ovarian syndrome, heart disease, and cancer. Let's deal with each of these in turn.

carbs and diabetes

Symptoms Of Diabetes

- Frequent trips to the restroom
- Continuous thirst
- Weight loss
- Nausea
- Easily tired
- Cravings for sweet foods
- Frequent gum, skin, vaginal, and urinary tract infections
- Blurred vision
- Pain in legs, feet, fingers
- Itching
- Drowsiness
- Cuts and bruises heal slowly

According to the American Diabetes Association, there are 18.2 million people in the U.S., or 6.3 percent of the population, who have diabetes. That's an estimated 13 million with a definite diagnosis of diabetes and 5.2 million people (or nearly one-third) unaware that they have the disease.

What is diabetes?

There are two main types of diabetes:
- Type I diabetes which is also known as insulin-dependent diabetes or juvenile onset diabetes
- Type II diabetes, also referred to as non-insulin dependent diabetes or middle aged onset diabetes

Type I diabetes

This usually appears before you reach the age of forty and is often called juvenile onset diabetes. This type of diabetes develops if the body cannot produce any insulin. As previously explained, insulin is produced in an organ of our body called the pancreas. In type I diabetes, the immune system attacks the cells of the pancreas so that eventually it can't produce any insulin. So after every meal, the levels of blood glucose remains high while, paradoxically, the body cells are starving of glucose because insulin isn't there to help the cells take up glucose from the blood.

This type of diabetes can therefore only be treated by regular insulin injections, which help the body cells take up glucose from the blood. Insulin can't be taken orally because it is made up of protein and will be digested by the enzymes in the gut and therefore render it useless.

Type II or middle aged onset diabetes

This is the more common condition and accounts for 80–90 percent of all cases diagnosed in the U.S. and U.K.

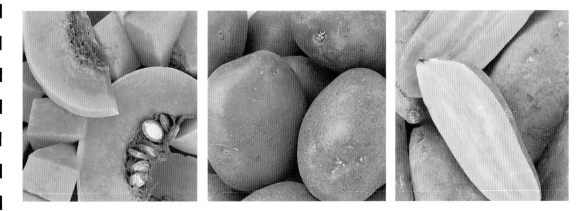

This type of diabetes usually appears after the age of 40 and develops either because the body can't make enough insulin or that the insulin produced doesn't work properly—meaning that the body cells, including our fat cells, become resistant to the presence of insulin (a term known as insulin resistance) so that the body cells are slow to take up glucose. This type of diabetes tends to run in families, and people with type II diabetes also tend to become overweight and obese because they tend to overeat. The theory is that the larger the fat cells become, the more resistant they become to insulin and the more obese the person. Obesity makes insulin resistance worse, which in turn makes obesity worse.

The choice of treatment for type II diabetes depends on the severity and is either by:
- diet and exercise alone, or
- diet, exercise, and tablets, or
- diet, exercise, and insulin injections.

Complications

Having diabetes means that there is an increased risk of developing complications such as heart disease, kidney disease, eye problems, nerve damage, and feet and skin problems. This is why it's so important to take good care of your heath and make healthy dietary and lifestyle choices if you do have diabetes.

Carbs, GI, and the diabetes connection

One of the most important applications of the GI scoring system is in the area of diabetes. If you remember from previous chapters, a higher intake of low rather than high GI foods results in starches and sugars being digested and absorbed more slowly into the bloodstream? Well, this has particularly important implications for people with diabetes who need to regulate their blood sugar levels.

Numerous studies have looked at the relationship between the GI factor and diabetes. In the U.S., a Nurses Health Study followed the diets of 65,173 women over a period of 6 years. The results showed that those who were diagnosed with diabetes and who had a high intake of cereal fiber together with a low glycemic load of foods reduced their risk of developing diabetes by two and a half times compared to those who ate high GI foods and low amounts of cereal fiber.

A six-year Health Professionals Follow Up study of 42,759 men found that the risk of developing diabetes was related to a combination of high glycemic load and low cereal. High glycemic load together with a low intake of cereal fiber increased the risk of type II diabetes by two fold compared to those with a high intake of cereal fiber and low glycemic load.

The Iowa's Health Study looking at 35,988 women over a period of six years found that the higher the consumption of total grains, wholegrains, total fiber, and cereal fiber was associated with a lower incidence of type II diabetes. The risk of diabetes was reduced by 21 percent in women eating more than 17 servings of wholegrains a week compared to those eating less than three servings a week. Women who ate more than 33 servings of wholegrains a week reduced their risk by even more (33 percent) compared to those eating less than 13 servings a week. Findings from these studies suggest that eating between 2–4 servings of wholegrains a day can decrease the risk of developing diabetes.

What can I eat?

Many people think that it's the end of the world if they have been diagnosed with diabetes and that they have to follow a special diet or give up cookies and candy for the rest of their life. According to the American Diabetic Association, people with diabetes can still enjoy a wide variety of foods as part of a balanced diet. When making dietary choices remember the following:

Choose a healthy balanced diet According to the American Diabetes Association, no single food will give you all the nutrients you need, so good nutrition always means eating a variety of foods.

Eat more starches The American Diabetes Association message is for everyone to "eat more wholegrains, beans, starchy vegetables (corn, potatoes, winter squash) because starches contain very little fat, saturated fat, or cholesterol. Foods with carbohydrates will raise your blood glucose more quickly than meats and fats, but they are the healthiest foods for you." They offer the following tips on how to include additional wholegrains, beans, and starchy vegetables into your diet:

- In a meatloaf or meatball recipe, substitute grain, such as oatmeal, bulgur, or brown rice, for some of the meat.

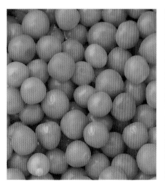

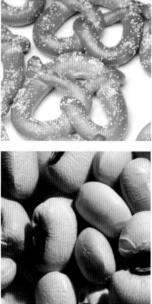

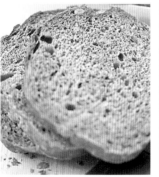

- Add noodles, peas, or beans to vegetable soup.
- Prepare a hearty bean or pea soup. Eat some and divide the rest into individual portions. You can then store the soup in the freezer for a quick meal.
- When you're cooking grains, make enough for extra servings. Then toss them on salads, into soups or casseroles, or reheat them as leftovers.
- Eat wholegrain cold cereal as a snack and pack the small boxes for snacks on the run.
- Add a can of chickpeas (garbanzo beans) or kidney beans to a salad, tomato sauce, or a three-bean salad.
- Treat yourself to great tasting wholegrain bread with meals, for a snack, or as the main course at breakfast.
- Add crunch to a salad or casserole with fat-free tortilla or potato chips.
- Have pretzels or light (in fat) popcorn for a snack.
- Buy breads with at least 2–3g of fiber and hot and cold cereals with at least 4g of fiber per serving.
(Source: www.diabetes.org)

Eat the GI way The Glycemic Index was initially developed as a research tool for planning diabetic diets (see Chapter 4 for more details). The Food and Agriculture Organization and the World Health Organization recommend low GI foods to be used. Choosing wholegrain, unrefined foods with more fiber or other low GI foods, such as whole fruits, milk, and beans, means that a slower rise in blood sugar is produced and helps to contribute to the control and regulation of blood glucose.

Try and cut down on the fat you eat Especially animal (saturated) fats. Too much fat or cholesterol may increase the chances of developing heart disease, so heart-smart choices include switching to monounsaturated fats such as those coming from olive oil and rapeseed oil. Not only is this healthier for your heart, but eating less fat and fatty foods will also help you to lose weight.

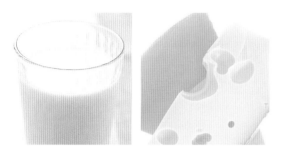

Follow these top tips to help you cut down on cholesterol and fat:

- Choose low-fat foods wherever you can, such as skim or low-fat milk, reduced-fat cheese, diet margarine, and yogurt.
- Choose lean cuts of meat and remove visible fat either before or after cooking
- Steam or broil instead of deep frying or cooking with oil or other fats. This will help you cut down on the amount of fat you eat and also the number of calories you consume.
- Limit the number of eggs you eat to no more than three or four a week

Eat more fruit and vegetables every day Choose a wide variety, the more colorful the better. This will provide you with all the vitamins and fiber you need for a healthy balanced diet and there are plenty of reasons to color-code your diet. For example, cancer and heart disease are thought to be attributed to the effects of free radicals. Free radicals are the natural by-products of biochemical reactions that are produced during metabolism and by the body's immune system. Pollution, radiation, pesticides, cigarette smoke, and herbicides can also be a source of free radicals. If these toxic agents are allowed to build up in the body, they can damage the structure and insides of our cells. If our bodies can't repair the damage, these cells are more likely to develop cancer. In the case of heart disease, free radicals can play a part in the formation of deposits in our blood vessels. If these deposits are left to accumulate they can cause the blood vessels to narrow and thus affect blood supply to the heart. If the blood vessels become completely blocked, blood won't be able to flow through to the heart, which can eventually lead to a heart attack. Fruits and vegetables contain phytochemicals (*phyto* meaning plants) such as carotenoids and flavonoids. These have antioxidant properties, which mean they have the ability to fight off or neutralize free radicals in the body.

Control the amount of sugar/sugary foods you eat
The FAO/WHO recommends not more than 10 percent of energy from sucrose. This doesn't mean you need to eat a completely sugar-free diet. For example, sugar can be used as an ingredient in foods and in baking as part of a healthy diet. However, make sure you choose either sugar-free, low-sugar, or diet versions of sugary drinks, which can cause blood glucose levels to rise quickly.

Use less salt That's because eating large quantities of salt and salty foods can raise your blood pressure. Having high blood pressure is linked to an increased risk of stroke and heart disease. Many of the foods we eat contain salt, often you can taste it in bacon, canned meats, or pickles, but a lot of the salt we eat is "hidden," for example, processed foods like cold cuts, prepared foods, cheeses, salad dressings, and canned soups. Try experimenting with recipes by adding herbs, spices, and lemon juice instead of salt. Choosing more fresh and unprocessed foods and banishing the salt shaker from the table will also help you keep your salt levels down.

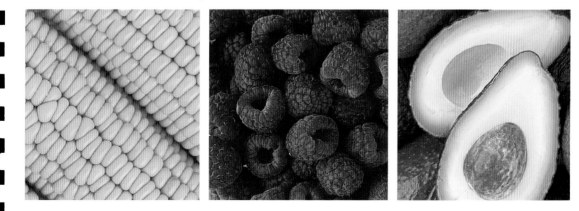

Pantry basics for flavor
Allspice
Basil
Bay leaves
Celery salt
Chili powder
Chilies
Cinnamon
Cloves
Cumin
Curry powder
Dill
Mustard
Fenugreek
Garlic
Ginger
Italian seasoning
Lemon grass
Low sodium soy sauce or low sodium teriyaki sauce or shoyu
Low sodium chicken, vegetable, or beef broth
Nutmeg
Onion powder
Oregano
Paprika
Parsley
Peppercorns
Rosemary
Sesame seeds
Thyme
Tomatoes (canned)
Worcestershire sauce
Vinegar (white wine, red wine, or balsamic)

Drink alcohol in moderation The American Diabetes Association guidelines suggest that we should not consume more than two alcoholic drinks a day if you are a man and one drink a day if you are a woman. You also need to check that your medications don't require you to avoid alcohol, and not to drink on an empty stomach. A drink is an equivalent to a 5 oz. glass of wine, a 12 oz. glass of light beer, or 1–1 1/2 oz. of 80 percent proof distilled spirits.

Losing weight If you're overweight losing the extra pounds will help you control diabetes. This will also reduce the risk of heart disease, high blood pressure, and stroke. Losing a small amount and keeping it off will help with blood glucose control and improve overall health.

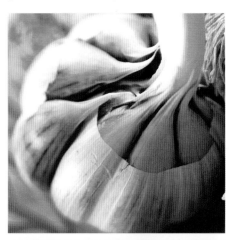

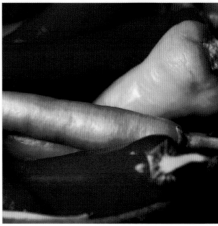

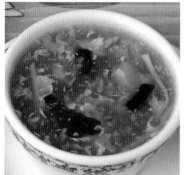
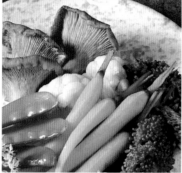

Healthy options at meal times Eating regularly and spreading your carb intake evenly throughout the day is an important factor in controlling your blood glucose levels. Here are some tips on what to choose for your meals throughout the day:

- High fiber wholegrain cereals with skim or low-fat milk.
- Unsweetended fruit juice, fresh, dried, or canned fruit in a juice.
- Wholegrain breads or toast instead of white, refined breads.
- Reduced sugar jelly, or marmalade or pure fruit spreads.
- Bran muffins.
- Seasonal foods make great economical choices as well as delicious snacks throughout the day.
- Eliminate the French fries and opt for boiled, baked, or steamed potatoes instead.
- Choose fresh fruit or low-fat yogurts as desserts.
- Eat an extra portion of vegetables or salad with your dinner.
- Soups make great appetizers, so try to choose clear broth, bouillon, or consommé when eating out.
- Drizzle salads with low-calorie dressings to keep the fat and calorie contents down.

Source: Adapted from The Cleveland Clinic website www.lifeclinic.com

For great tips and general information about diabetes, look at the American Diabetes Association website www.diabetes.org or the Cleveland Clinic website as above. For help in planning your carbs intake, always ask your dietician or doctor for help.

Typical daily plans for people with diabetes

Main meal containing 45g of carbohydrates

3 oz. chicken breast or broiled salmon or lean beef slices

$2/3$ cup rice

1 cup broccoli

salad with low-fat, low-carbohydrate dressing

1 cup of low-fat milk or a small roll

Breakfast containing 75g of carbohydrates

4 pancakes (4 in. diameter)

2 tbsp. regular maple syrup

$3/4$ cup of blueberries

Main meal containing 75g of carbohydrates

$1^1/2$ cups of spaghetti with $1/2$ cup of sauce

2 meatballs

Parmesan cheese

1 cup of green beans

Salad with low-fat, low-carbohydrate dressing

1 oz. slice of garlic bread

Water with lemon

Artificial sweeteners—what is their role in a diabetic diet?

Since sugar counts as a carb, it is not considered a "free food," and needs to be worked into a meal plan for someone with diabetes—ideally during consultation with a dietician. If and when you choose to eat foods containing sugar, you need to substitute them for carbohydrate foods in your meal plan.

The nutrition facts label on packaged foods will tell you, for example, how many grams of total carbohydrates, fiber, and sugars are in a serving of that food (as shown below). Artificial sweeteners are useful aids for those of us who want to limit the amount of sugar

we eat. There are two groups of artificial sweeteners:

Sugar alcohols This group includes sorbitol, mannitol, and xylitol. Sorbitol is the most widely used in products such as sugar-free gum or dietetic foods. Sugar alcohols yields three calories per gram. Because sugar alcohols have a different chemical structure to simple sugars, they are not readily broken down by bacteria in our mouths and so the great news is that they are not cariogenic, in other words they don't promote dental caries. Furthermore, they don't spike blood sugar levels and so are used in dietetic foods. The real disadvantage is their laxative effect. This is caused because they are not absorbed readily in the gut so if you eat large amounts of sugar alcohols (50g or more a day), you are likely to develop diarrhea.

Alternative sweeteners This group includes saccharin, aspartame, and acesulfame K and have been approved by the U.S. Food and Drink Administration as being safe to use. These low calorie sweeteners make food taste sweet and don't spike blood sugar levels. They also don't count as a carbohydrate:

- Saccharin was first made in the late 1800s. Today it is widely available and is used in both hot and cold foods and in soft drinks to make them sweeter. Saccharin is 300 times sweeter than sucrose. Questions still linger about whether saccharin may cause cancer in humans, and though the sweetener is still widely used, it carries a label that warns of its potential risks.

Nutritional information label	
Serving Size 1 Cup (228g)	
Serving Per Container 2	
	% Daily Value*
Calories 250	
Calories From Fat 110	
Total Fat 12g	18%
Saturated Fat 3g	15%
Trans Fat 1.5g	
Cholesterol 30mg	10%
Sodium 470mg	20%
Total Carbohydrate 31g	10%
Dietary Fiber 0g	0%
Sugars 5g	
Protein 5g	
Vitamin A	4%
Vitamin C	2%
Calcium	20%
Iron	4%

*Percent Daily Values are based on a 2,000 calorie diet.

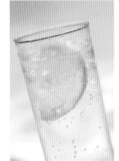
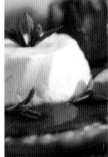

- Aspartame (NutraSweet or Equal) was first made available in 1981. Aspartame is made up of the amino acids (protein building blocks), phenylalanine, and aspartic acid. Aspartame is 200 times sweeter than sucrose and so only very small amounts are needed to make foods taste sweet. This alternative sweetener is used in sodas, gelatin-containing desserts, and chewing gum. Because aspartame is made up of amino acids, its chemical structure is changed when heated, so it tends not to be used in products that need to be cooked. Some people have a rare disease called phenylketonuria (PKU), which means they cannot metabolize phenylalanine properly and toxic by-products build up in the body and lead to mental retardation. This means that phenylketonurics cannot eat or drink anything containing this amino acid. So products containing aspartame have to carry the warning: "Phenylketonurics: Contains Phenylalanine." Aspartame hasn't been linked with cancer but some people have reported sensitivities or adverse reactions to it including headaches, dizziness, seizures, and nausea.
- Acesulfame potassium (Sweet One, Sunett, or acesulfame-K). The FDA approved this sweetener for use in 1998. Acesulfame-K is 200 times sweeter than sucrose and is used in chewing gum, gelatins, non-dairy creamers, yogurt, puddings, frozen desserts, syrups, toppings, and baked goods. It can also be used for all baking and cooking needs. Often you can't achieve the same texture in baked products if you use it instead of sucrose. Like other alternative sweeteners, you may need to add some table sugar to improve texture.

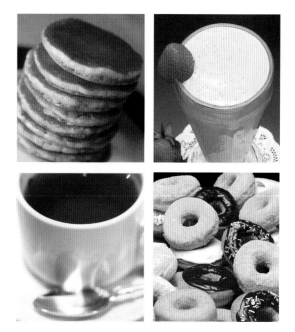

- Sucralose (Splenda) is the newest kid on the block. Sucralose can be used anywhere sugar can be used. It is actually made from table sugar, but cannot be digested. It is between 400 and 800 times sweeter than sucrose. It also does not affect blood sugar levels, so is suitable for diabetics.

All of these artificial sweeteners may help people who have diabetes to control their sugar intake without losing the sweetness they enjoy in foods. They are also a helpful aid to those of us who want to lose weight, reduce our calories, and stick to a healthy meal plan.

carbs and hypoglycemia

It is not uncommon to hear people saying that they feel "hypo," but what exactly is this feeling and why does it happen? Hypoglycemia is a condition that can develop if your blood sugar levels drops too low. Many believe that this only happens to diabetics but you certainly do not have to have diabetes to experience low sugar levels. For example, the condition can be triggered if you do any of the following:

- Delay or skip a meal
- Eat too little food at any meal
- Exercise more than usual
- Drink alcohol
- Take too much medicine for diabetes

People suffering from hypoglycemia can experience any number, or various combinations, of symptoms. The physical effects can often include feeling shaky, nervous, tired, sweaty, cold, irritable, or headachy. If you think that your blood glucose is too low then health experts recommend that you should do one or all of the following things:

- Eat regular meals, ensuring that you have a sustaining intake of carbs.
- Make sure that there is protein, fat, and fiber in every meal that you eat in order to prevent major swings in your blood sugar levels.
- Eat complex carbs which should include plenty of foods that contain insoluble fiber.

- Eat snacks containing small amounts of protein, such as half a lean-meat sandwich made using whole-wheat bread together with a glass of skim or low-fat milk.
- Avoid meals or snacks of that consist solely of simple carbs.
- Consume only moderate amounts of caffeine and alcohol.

carbs and lactose intolerance

As discussed in Chapter 1, lactose is a simple carb which is made up of two sugars joined together—a disaccharide. This particular sugar is commonly found in the milk of animals such as cows, goats, and sheep, and also in human milk. Lactose has to be broken down into its constituent sugars before the body can absorb it. This process occurs in the gut by the action of an enzyme called lactase. I will explain some of the terminology before we go any further. Lactose intolerance refers to a number of symptoms such as bloating, abdominal pain, flatulence, diarrhea, or constipation. Lactose maldigestion occurs in many population groups where the practice of milk drinking declines after infancy. Decrease in the lactase enzyme activity usually occurs between the ages of two and 20 years in the majority of the world's population. While people with lactose intolerance often develop abdominal symptoms after eating foods containing lactose, those who are lactose maldigesters do not develop these types of symptoms. Most

people in the developed world retain the ability to produce the enzyme lactase because they continue drinking milk and eating dairy products throughout their childhood and into adulthood. The reason why people who have lactose maldigestion don't suffer from abdominal symptoms after eating lactose-containing foods is because they retain enough levels of the enzyme lactase to digest moderate amounts of lactose.

Who might have lactose intolerance?
It is not uncommon for lactose intolerance to occur temporarily, particularly in infants as a response to viral gastrienteritis or in adults as a response to infection or disease in the part of the gut that produces lactase.

There is a proven genetic predisposition to lactose maldigestion; it is more common in South East Asia, India, the Middle East, certain parts of Africa and areas of the world which have not traditionally supported the development of dairying. The prevalence of lactose intolerance in non-white races is about 5 percent in children under four years old and increases to around 33 percent by 13 years. In contrast the prevalence is very low in Caucasian children. According to the National Institute of Health, between 30–50 million Americans are lactose intolerant. While up to 75 percent of the black African community and more than 90 percent of the Asian community are intolerant to lactose. In the UK, the prevalence of lactose maldigestion is about 5 percent and about 2 percent of the population have lactose intolerance.

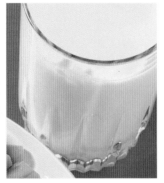

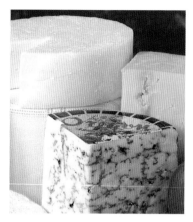

Temporary lactose intolerance can occur in infants as a result of gastro-enteritis; this is usually treated with a complete withdrawal of milk, which is replaced by a glucose and electrolyte mixture.

How is lactose intolerance diagnosed?
The most common tests used are the lactose tolerance test and the hydrogen breath test. These tests are usually done on an outpatient basis, usually at a hospital or clinic. Here is a brief summary of the processes:

Lactose tolerance test After a night of fasting before the test, the individual is given a liquid that contains lactose. Several blood samples are taken over a two-hour period to measure the person's blood glucose levels. This gives an indication of how well the body is able to digest or break down lactose. They are able to use this as an indicator as when lactose reaches the gut, the lactase enzyme breaks it down into glucose and galactose. Glucose enters the bloodstream and raising blood glucose levels. If lactose is completely digested, blood glucose levels don't rise and a diagnosis of lactose intolerance is made.

Hydrogen breath test This measures the amount of hydrogen in a person's breath. Under normal circumstances, very little hydrogen is produced but if lactose is incompletely broken down, it passes down to the colon where it is fermented by bacteria, producing hydrogen. This hydrogen passes to the lungs and is exhaled, after being absorbed from the gut and passing through the bloodstream. During the test, the individual is given a lactose containing drink and the breath is analyzed at regular intervals. Raised levels of hydrogen in the breath indicate that lactose is incompletely digested.

(Neither the lactose tolerance or hydrogen breath tests are given to infants or very young children because giving them large doses of lactose can be dangerous for them if they are found to be intolerant.)

Double blind placebo controlled food challenge This is considered to be the gold standard for the diagnosis of lactose intolerance. These challenges are performed in a way that neither the individual nor the person performing the test knows the identity of the food given or which substance is the placebo. Dehydrated or dried powdered food is administered in either gelatin capsules or disguised in a food carrier, for example, an apple or vegetable puree or lentil soup. The placebo is either a gelatine capsule or the food carrier with nothing added. A small sample of the food is usually administered and the dose is doubled at intervals and continued until the patient has obvious symptoms. There is always a risk of inducing anaphylactic shock, so these tests should always be conducted in a hospital where this can be dealt with if necessary.

Calcium
Milk and other dairy products are a major source of nutrients in our diet, particularly calcium. Calcium is essential for the growth and repair of bones throughout life. In the middle and later years, a deficiency of calcium may lead to thin, fragile bones that break easily—a condition known as osteoporosis. For both children and adults with lactose intolerance, it is important to get enough calcium in a diet that includes little or no milk.

How do you improve intolerance?

In most cases, lactose intolerance can be improved. Below is some brief advice and information on handling the condition:

- Adjusting the amount eaten at any one time or by eating foods which contain lactose as part of a meal.
- Eliminating milk and dairy products completely is often unnecessary and may lead to deficiencies of certain nutrients found naturally in these products, such as calcium, riboflavin, and vitamin B12.
- Hard cheeses (like Cheddar) and fermented milk products (such as, yogurt, and yogurt drinks). Those with live cultures are better tolerated because the bacteria used in yogurt carry their own form of lactase and the presence of

this enzyme performs the same function as human lactase. As a result yogurt tends to be better tolerated than milk.

- For those people with a severe lactase deficiency, a yeast derived form of lactase is available that can be added to milk either during processing in the dairy (known as lactose-reduced milk) or by the consumer. The lactase breaks down lactose into its component sugars before it is actually consumed.
- Many non-dairy foods are high in calcium and don't contain any lactose, such as green vegetables and fish with soft, edible bones, such as salmon and sardines. (See table 1 for examples.)

Other dairy foods, which are better tolerated, contain small amounts of lactose and are rich in calcium (see table 2).

1. High-calcium, non-dairy foods

Food	Portion	Calcium	Lactose
Calcium fortified orange juice	1 cup	308–344	0
Sardines, canned with bones	3oz.	270	0
Salmon, canned with bones	3oz.	205	0
Calcium fortified soymilk	1 cup	200	0
Broccoli, raw	1 cup	90	0
Orange	1 medium	50	0
Pinto beans, cooked	1/2 cup	40	0
Tuna, canned	3oz.	10	0
Lettuce leaves	1/2 cup	10	0

Reference: National Digestive Diseases Information Clearinghouse, National Institute of Health

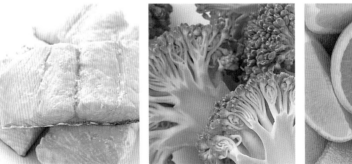
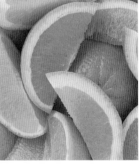

2. Low-lactose dairy foods

Food	Portion	Calcium	Lactose
Unflavored yogurt, low-fat	1 cup	415	5
Milk, reduced-fat	1 cup	295	11
Swiss cheese	1oz.	270	1
Ice cream	1/2 cup	85	6
Plain cottage cheese	1/2 cup	75	2–3

Reference: National Digestive Diseases Information Clearinghouse, National Institute of Health

Hidden lactose

There are many prepared foods which contain lactose, and people with a low tolerance to lactose should be aware that the following foods also contain small amounts of "hidden" lactose:

- bread and other baked products
- some breakfast cereals
- instant potatoes, soups, and drinks
- canned soups and stews
- some margarines and fat spreads
- luncheon or other canned meat products
- salad dressings and marinades
- candies and other confectionery
- ready mixes for pancakes, cookies, cakes, etc.
- powdered meal replacements

Lactose-free foods

- Lactaid 100 milk (completely lactose-free milk—you can also buy other types of Lactaid milk which are reduced in lactose, such as, non-fat to one percent fat Lactaid milk is 70 percent lactose reduced, non-fat calcium-fortified Lactaid milk is fortified with 500mg calcium per cup of milk and is 70 percent lactose reduced)
- Soy milk
- Fresh fruit and vegetables
- Wheat-based breads
- Rice cakes
- Graham crackers
- All types of wholegrains, rice, pasta, oats, barley, bulgur wheat
- Plain lamb, beef, pork, veal, poultry, shellfish, fish, eggs, pulses, beans
- Canned fish, for example, tuna, salmon
- Non-dairy creamers
- Vegetable oils
- Gelatin
- Fruit ice
- Fruit and vegetable juices
- Plain coffee or tea
- Bouillon
- Broth
- Honey
- Preserves

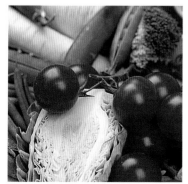
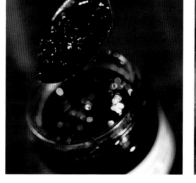
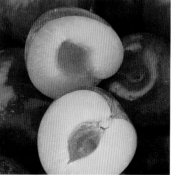

Label Savvy

Know your food labels by looking for the following terms:

- milk
- lactose
- whey
- curds
- dry milk solids
- non-fat milk powder
- some types of non-prescription and also prescription drugs, birth control pills, and indigestion tablets contain lactose

If you would like to know more about lactose intolerance, you can contact the following organizations for further information:

National Digestive Diseases Information Clearinghouse (www.digestive.niddk.nih.gov)

American Dietetic Association (www.eatright.org)

International Foundation for Functional Gastrointestinal Disorders (www.iffgd.org)

Typical daily plan for a lactose-free diet

Breakfast: High-fiber cereal or oatmeal with calcium-fortified soy milk or wholegrain toast. Coffee or tea with calcium fortified soy milk

Lunch: Whole-wheat pasta salad with canned tuna, canned corn, and vinaigrette dressing, or sandwich made with whole-wheat pita bread stuffed with tomatoes, hummus, and cucumber. Canned or fresh fruit. Water, fruit juice

Dinner: Pork and vegetable stir fry with steamed brown rice. Soy yogurt with fresh fruit

Snacks: Fresh fruit, crackers with salsa.

Remember
You should always consult your doctor or dietician for advise about planning or starting a suitable diet if you think you may be lactose intolerant.

carbs and the pms connection

It's the same story every month: one or more weeks of agonizing stomach cramps, aching back, bad moods, and bloating, and an insatiable craving for mountains of candy and fries. Does this sound like you? Well you're certainly not alone. It's estimated that eight out of ten women experience some or all of these symptoms every single month before their periods arrive. In fact, according to the American College of Obstetricians and Gynaecologists around 40 percent of women of childbearing age experience physical and emotional symptoms of pre-menstrual syndrome (PMS) that are severe enough to affect their daily routines and activities.

PMS describes a whole host of physical and mental problems that affect women before and during our menstrual cycle. Some also suffer additionally from water retention, mood swings, irritability, depression, anxiety, acne, constipation, diarrhea, and tender

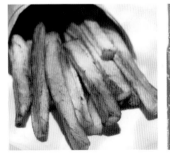
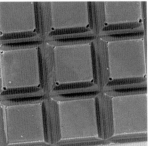

breasts. Unfortunately, no one knows why women suffer from PMS and the bad news continues because there's no proven way to cure it either. So are we doomed for the rest of our lives?

Millions of women have found that they can manage their PMS better by simply changing their diet. This is because certain foods affect the levels of a specific hormone called estrogen. Furthermore, being physically active and exercising has also been found to help alleviate painful stomach cramps *and* boost your mood. This is due to the fact that when we exercise, "happy" hormones called endorphins are released by the brain, which improve our mood and help us to relax.

Where do carbs fit into the story?

The majority of women who have PMS say they crave simple carbohydrates, particularly sugar, right before their periods. Many of us indulge this craving, eating often unlimited quantities of chocolate, chips, pastry, candy, cookies, and breads. A study published in the *Journal of Reproductive Medicine* showed that women who tended to eat sugar-rich foods such as candy, fruit juice, and alcoholic beverages had the most severe PMS symptoms. As a consequence of studies such as these,

many women adopt strict carb curfews. But is this the right approach?

No, say doctors Judith J. and Richard J. Wurtman. The husband and wife team based at the Massachusetts Institute of Technology in Boston, in the U.S. believe that women suffering from PMS *shouldn't* in fact avoid carbs. Their research showed that meals and snacks rich in carbohydrates substantially improved depression, tension, anger, and other symptoms of pre-menstrual syndrome (PMS) in two groups of women who took part in their study.

PMS, according to the MIT researchers, shares certain similarities with Seasonal Affective Disorder (SAD), a mild form of depression which occurs during Fall and winter. Apparently, people with SAD show significant improvements in their mood after eating meals rich in carbs and low in protein. The MIT researchers even go as far as to suggest that cravings for carbohydrates reported by women who suffer from PMS isn't the result of any nutritional deficiencies rather that it's a brain deficiency of serotonin (a hormone that influences our mood). One way you can make serotonin is by eating carbohydrates.

Sixty participants took part in the MIT study, and

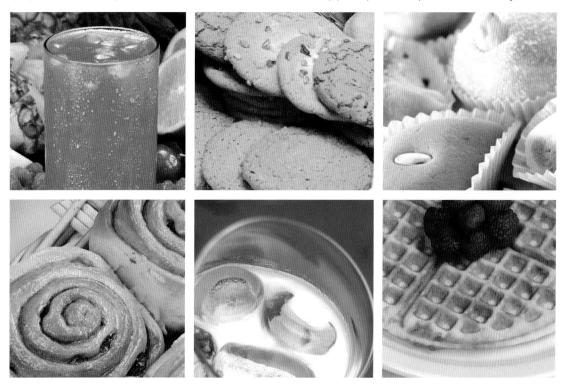

consisted of two study groups of women with and without PMS. The study showed that consumption of a carbohydrate-rich, protein-poor test meal during the late phase of the menstrual cycle improved depression, tension, anger, confusion, sadness, fatigue, alertness, and calmness scores as measured on standard tests for PMS patients. No effects were seen among control subjects.

In another study published in the *Journal of Obstetrics and Gynaecology* in 1995, women with PMS given a high-carb, low-protein drink scored lower in the depression index indicating

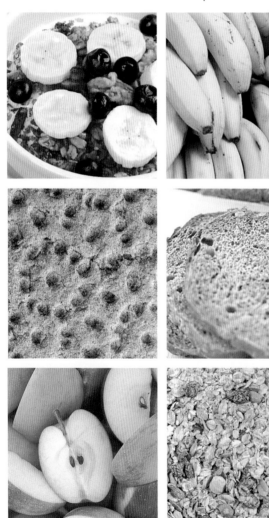

that their mood was improved with intake of carbohydrate. These findings are supported by another study, which showed those women given meals rich in carbohydrate, but low in protein combined with regular exercise showed a "decline in menstrual distress." The researchers concluded that this type of "treatment" only seems to work among women in luteal phase of their menstrual cycle. Women without PMS didn't demonstrate any improvements in mood after a carb-rich, low-protein meal, indicating that carbohydrates function in different way for individuals with and without PMS. The research suggests that carbohydrates exert an effect on the level of the hormone progesterone during luteal phase, thereby producing an antidepressant effect on PMS.

Carb cures for PMS

So, our craving for candy and other things sweet and high in fat are our body's way of telling us that we need more serotonin. But are these fatty and sugary treats the best way to relieve PMS symptoms? Well, high-fat and high-sugar foods are certainly the quickest way of raising serotonin levels but *stop* before you grab your nearest packet of Oreos or chocolate covered ice cream bar. These refined carbs will also raise your blood sugar levels quickly and what goes up will come down. In this case blood sugar levels will decline rapidly, making you hungry again! Happily, this is where our heroine of the story again comes in—complex carbs. Complex carbs will raise serotonin levels but at a much more sustainable levels, so when PMS cravings strike reach for a rye crispbread instead.

Top tips for staving off cravings

Eat small frequent meals Six small meals a day will do, this can help keep blood sugar levels stable and helps us to avoid cravings. Instead of eating more, you just eat smaller amounts more often.

Eat small complex carbs snacks every 3 hours Try wholegrain cereals, wholegrain crackers, bananas, apples, whole-wheat sandwiches, and rye crispbreads—though of course it will have to be half your normal quantities so you don't eat more than you would normally.

Drink 6–8 glasses of water a day This will reduce pre-menstrual bloating.

Here are some tips for controlling PMS itself:

- Eat complex carbohydrates, such as wholegrain breads, pasta, cereals, and fiber. Cut back on sugar and fat.

- Avoid salt for the last few days before your period to reduce bloating and fluid retention.
- Cut back on caffeine to feel less tense and irritable and to ease PMS breast soreness.
- Get moving with aerobic exercise.
- Get plenty of sleep.
- Regulate meals, bedtime, and exercise.
- If possible, try to schedule stressful events for the week after your period.

Knowing PMS is coming doesn't make it any easier to handle, but simple changes to your diet can really help.

carbs and polycystic ovarian syndrome

PCOS stands for Polycystic Ovarian Syndrome (PCOS), but it is sometimes referred to as polycystic ovaries or polycystic ovarian disease (PCOD). PCOS is thought to affect around five to 10 percent of all women and is one of the main causes of infertility.

What are the symptoms PCOS?
The symptoms vary from women to women and can include some or all of the following, which can all be compounded by weight gain:

- periods problems (absent, heavy, irregular)
- ovarian cysts
- excess facial and/or body hair
- hair loss (similar to the pattern baldness experienced by men)
- weight gain
- acne or excessively oily skin
- skin tags
- brown skin patches

- high cholesterol levels
- high blood pressure
- tiredness
- decreased sex drive
- excess "male" hormones, for example, androgens or testosterone
- infertility
- decrease in size of breasts
- enlarged ovaries or uterus

What is the cause of PCOS? The insulin connection
No one knows exactly what the cause of PCOS is but it is thought that PCOS is related to a problem with insulin. If you remember, the pancreas produces insulin after a meal allowing our body cells to take up glucose thus fulfilling our energy needs? Well, in PCOS it is thought that our body cells don't respond to normal amounts of insulin—what is known as insulin resistance. As a result the pancreas makes more insulin to try and compensate

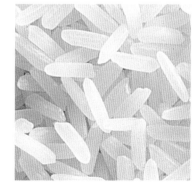
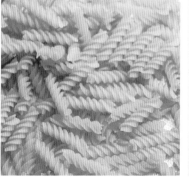
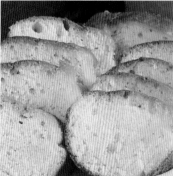

for this problem. High levels of insulin means an increased risk of developing type II diabetes, becoming overweight or obese, and the risk of heart disease. Additionally, high levels of insulin have the effect of stimulating our ovaries to make large amounts of androgens (male hormones like testosterone) which has the effect of preventing ovulation and therefore causing infertility.

Tests for PCOS

Usually your doctor will arrange for you to see an endocrinologist (someone specializing in hormones). They may suggest one or more tests. For example, blood tests that look at glucose, cholesterol levels, hormonal levels of testosterone compared with lutenizing hormone (LH), and follicle stimulating hormone (FSH). Ultrasound tests can check for the presence of ovarian cysts.

Diet and PCOS

People with PCOS often say that the symptoms are more severe when they gain weight and improve if they manage to lose some weight.

Some sufferers say that low-carb diets have helped them to lose weight and have therefore improved their symptoms. Health professionals recommend changing the types of carbs eaten, from refined to an unrefined diet containing more fresh vegetables and fruit. These changes would include:

- Swapping refined grains for wholegrains. So instead of white bread, white rice, white pasta, choose whole-wheat pasta, brown rice, or whole-wheat bread.
- Exchanging refined sugary cereals, sugary cereal bars, and donuts for wholegrain cereals.
- Drinking water or diet sodas instead of other sugary soft drinks.
- Replacing sugary foods such as cakes, cookies, muffins, and candy with sugar-free puddings and yogurt.
- Non-carb foods, such as protein-rich foods, have less of an effect on insulin and so can slow down the absorption of meals. Combine carbs, protein, and fats in each meal, for example reduced-fat peanut butter and whole-wheat bread.

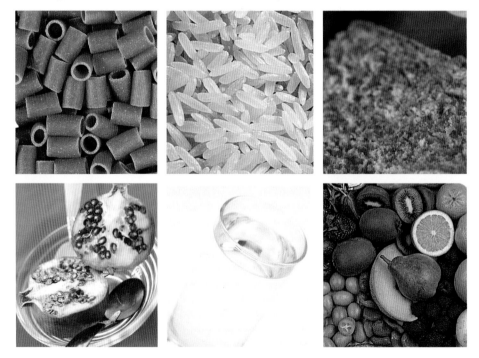

- Watch your portion sizes and have small frequent meals throughout the day to keep your insulin and blood sugar levels steady.
- If you are eating lots of carbs, particularly those low in fiber, always select smaller portions.

Move your body

Exercise is very important because it will help with weight loss and bring down insulin levels at the same time. If you haven't got time to go to the gym make sure you walk off your lunch or evening meal, or find an activity that is realistic for you, and aim for at around half an hour of exercise a day, at least three times a week.

For more information on PCOS, check out www.pcos.net or www.verity-pcos.org.uk

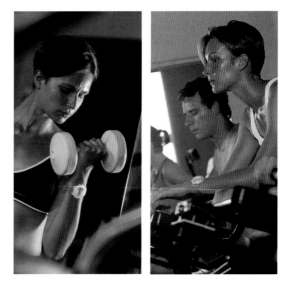

carbs and rheumatoid arthritis

You may have heard in the popular press that carbs cause arthritis. The proposed link between carbohydrates and rheumatoid arthritis was recently suggested in 2002 by researchers at the Brigham and Women's Hospital in Boston and also by the Harvard Medical School in Boston in 2002.

What is rheumatoid arthritis?

Rheumatoid arthritis is an autoimmune disease which currently affects around 2.1 million people across the U.S. and many more across the world. The disease occurs when the body's immune system starts attacking its own joints and cartilage.

The carb connection

A type of complex carbohydrate with the complex name of glycosaminoglycans (or GAGS) is found in the joints of our bones. Their job is to hold together the skin, fluid, cartilage, and other connective tissue. The Boston-based researchers proposed that the immune systems of people with rheumatoid arthritis target GAGs directly. Antibodies bind to GAGS and accumulate in the joints, thus causing the pain and inflammation associated with rheumatoid arthritis. While this theory is interesting, it is important to remember that although GAGS are complex carbs, they aren't related in any way to the carbs we eat in our diets.

carbs and heart disease

After cancer, heart disease is the major cause of death for women and men in both the U.S. There has been a lot in the press about how much and what type of carbs we should or shouldn't be eating for health and its implications for heart disease.

What is heart disease?

Symptoms of heart disease develop over many years and don't usually become obvious until we reach middle age.

Problems begin when the blood vessels to the heart narrow (due to the accumulation of cholesterol and small blood clots over time deposited on the blood vessel walls) reducing blood flow to the heart. Initially, this causes chest pain, called angina, usually after physical exertion.

Eventually one of the blood vessels may become totally blocked and stop blood supply to part of the heart. This leads to muscle damage due to the lack of

95

oxygen, which can cause a heart attack. If the damage is extensive, the heart may beat irregularly or stop altogether, which can be fatal. Risk factors for heart disease include smoking, being overweight or obese, being physically inactive, and having high blood pressure or high blood cholesterol.

The carb connection

Cereal grains such as whole-wheat, brown rice, whole oats, corn, and rye have been the staples of the world's diets for centuries. Rice in Asia and India, pasta in Italy, oats in

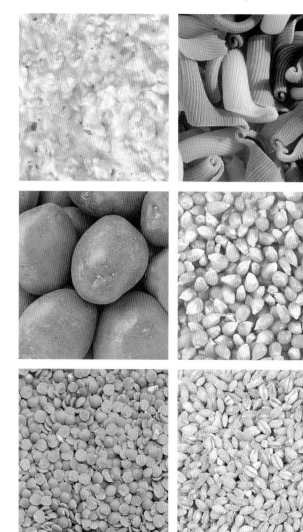

Scotland; and the range of grain products consumed around the world is truly amazing. As nations have become more industrialized, the majority of the grains eaten are in the refined form. As you know, removing the outer parts of the grains means that bran, nutrients such as vitamins E and B, selenium, zinc, copper, iron, fiber, and phytochemicals such as lignans and phytoestrogens, which protect against heart disease and cancers, are lost.

Numerous scientific studies have focused on the relationship between the risk of heart disease and carb intake. Dr. Pereira and his colleagues at the University of Minnesota collected data on 91,058 men and 245,186 women who took part in 10 studies in the U.S. and Europe. Each study looked at the foods eaten, and all studies measured the amount of fiber in their diets. Results were published in the Archives of Internal Medicine in 2002. During the 6–10 years of follow-up, 5,249 people were diagnosed with heart disease and 2,011 participants died. The study showed that for every 10g of cereal fiber eaten a day, the risk of death from heart disease was reduced by 25 percent. For every 10g of fruit fiber eaten daily, the risk dropped by 30 percent. Interestingly, no link was found between vegetable fiber and risk of heart disease. These results were independent of other factors that reduce the risk for heart disease, such as not smoking, exercising, and weight control. The authors concluded that the quality of the carbohydrate eaten was important, that is, fiber derived from wholegrains, unrefined cereals, fruit, and vegetables held the key to reducing the risk of heart disease.

The Iowa Women's Health Study followed 34,000 women aged between 55–64 years over a nine-year period. Results were published in 1998 in the *American Journal of Clinical Nutrition* and showed that women who ate at least one serving of wholegrain a day had a substantially lower risk of death from chronic heart disease (CHD) than those who didn't eat any.

The Nurses' Health Study, which followed a large group of women—over 80,000 in the U.S. over a period of up to 10 years—showed

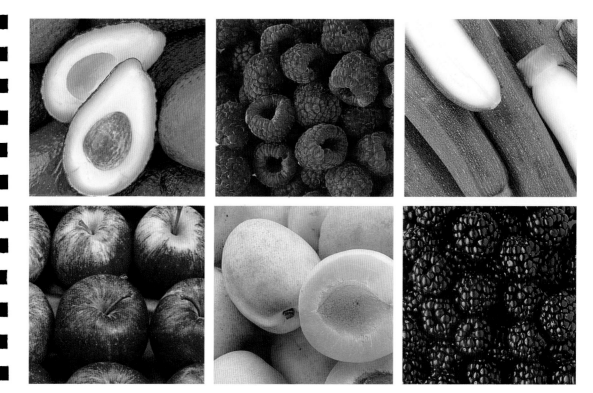

that higher fiber intake, particularly from cereals and wholegrain sources, such as dark breads, wholegrain breakfast cereals, popcorn, cooked oatmeal, wheatgerm, brown rice, and bran, reduces the risk of CHD.

Similarly, in the U.S. Health Professionals Study, which followed 43,757 male health professionals over a period of six years, found that for every 1g increase in fiber, there was a 29 percent decrease in the risk of developing coronary heart disease.

The Finnish ATBC (alpha-tocopherol, beta-carotene) cancer prevention study followed a group of male smokers aged between 50–60 years for over six years. The study showed that total dietary fiber intake, especially those coming form rye products, potatoes, vegetables, and fruits/berries, was proven to protect against developing CHD.

Where does GI fit into this story?

A diet that contains mainly low GI foods may help reduce the risk of heart disease. For example, a study published in the *American Journal of Clinical Nutrition* in 2000 looked at the diets of 75,521 women in the U.S. over a period of 10 years. It found that a high glycemic load (that is, a diet containing large quantities of high GI

foods, such as refined carbs) increases the risk of coronary heart disease. Subsequent studies have shown the same association concluding that by reducing the intake of high-glycemic beverages and replacing refined grain products and potatoes with minimally processed plant-based foods, such as whole grains, fruits, and vegetables, the incidence of CHD may be decreased in sedentary, overweight individuals.

Why do some carbs protect against CHD?

According to a joint report on *Carbohydrates in Human Nutrition*, by the Food and Agriculture Organization and the World Health Organization in 1997, there are a number of ways in which a high carbohydrate diet might be protective of against the development of cardiovascular disease:

- High-carb diets help to lower glucose and insulin levels, which in turn decreases the risk factors for cardiovascular disease.
- Carbs that are fermented in the colon produce substances called short chain fatty acids, which helps to regulate the way our liver handles glucose and insulin.

- Carbs provide micronutrients and phytochemicals, which tend to help keep the cardiovascular system healthy.
- Carbs tend to make us feel full and satisfied after we eat, so we are likely to eat fewer calories, therefore reducing ours chances of becoming overweight or obese.

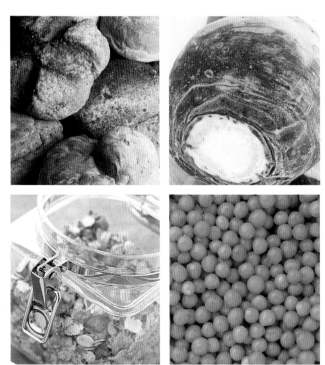

Take home points

After examining scientific evidence about the relationship between fiber intake and risk for coronary heart disease, the United States Food and Drug Administration (FDA) now allows food products which contain more than 51 percent wholegrains (including whole-wheat) to show the following health claim, that, "Diets rich in whole grains and other plant foods and low in total fat, saturated fats and cholesterol may reduce the risk of heart disease and some cancers."

The American Heart Association's guidelines for a healthy heart include the following advice relating to our carb intake:

- Eat a variety of fruits and vegetables. Choose five or more servings per day.
- Eat a variety of grain products, including whole grains. Choose six or more servings per day.
- Limit your intake of foods high in calories or low in nutrition.

(See their website for the full list of recommendations: www.americanheart.org)

Heart-smart choices for grains and cereal

Next time you go grocery shopping, make heart-smart choices by using the following guide to help you:

- For breads choose whole-grain, whole-wheat, mixed grain breads and English muffins, wholemeal pita breads, wholemeal flat bread, wholemeal crumpets, and wholegrain crispbreads.
- For hot or cold cereals choose wholegrain, whole-wheat, or high-fiber breakfast cereals, granola, or oats. (Granola-type cereals can be high in fat so check the label).
- For rice or pasta choose brown rice, whole-wheat pasta, or wild rice. Other starchy wholegrains include bulgur, quinoa, millet, flaxseeds.
- For starchy vegetables choose potatoes, corn, lima beans, green peas, winter squash, sweet potatoes.
- For soups choose chicken noodle, minestrone tomato-based seafood, onion chowders, and split pea.

One serving of grains equals
1 slice bread, or
1/4 cup nugget or bud-type cereal
1/2 cup hot cereal
1 cup flaked cereal
1 cup cooked rice or pasta
1/4 to 1/2 cup starchy vegetables
1 cup low-fat soup

carbs and cancer

There are many factors involved in the development of cancer, some are related to family history while others are related to lifestyle and diet.

What is cancer?

Our body is made up of small building blocks called cells. Dead, worn down, or damaged cells need to be replaced by new ones. New cells are also made during growth, for example, during adolescence, pregnancy, or infancy. Normally, the body controls the growth of new cells but sometimes abnormal or faulty cells are produced which don't function properly. Cancer of the cells may develop if these "faulty" cells aren't destroyed because they can multiply at a rapid rate spreading to other cells and different parts of the body.

How do carbs protect against cancer?

Fiber The protective effects of high-fiber foods against cancer of the colon were proposed back in the 1970s. A scientist called Burkitt suggested that an increased intake of refined cereals, protein, fat, and sugar were the culprits behind the rise in the incidences of cancer. Health experts believe that it is likely that fiber and various phytochemicals work together to protect against cancer. Most research has focused its attention on fiber and the various ways it may affect cancer risk. Researchers have suggested that fiber decreases the risk of cancer because it has the following effects.

- Increases the bulk of our stools.
- Decreases transit time of waste products through the colon, therefore allowing less opportunity for toxic compounds to remain in contact with its cells.
- Binds toxic compounds and so aids their elimination through the gut.
- Prevents insulin resistance.

It is now widely accepted that insoluble fibers such as those coming from wholegrains and cereals protect against cancer of the colon. Wholegrains contain carbohydrates, which can be fermented by the bacteria in our gut into protective substances called short chain fatty acids. These acids have been shown to reduce the activity of certain factors that cause cancers. In addition, grains and cereals contain a wide range of phytochemicals, which may inhibit the production of abnormal cells and so may suppress the growth of cancerous cells.

Fruit and vegetables Numerous scientific studies have shown that eating lots of fruit and vegetables may reduce the chance of developing some cancers such as lung and colon cancer. This may be because fruit and vegetables, which are valuable sources of soluble fiber, contain compounds called antioxidants. These antioxidants are like our knights in shining armor, protecting our body cells from being damaged. Antioxidants from fruit and vegetables include:

- *Carotenes (vegetable form of vitamin A) and vitamin A*: Numerous studies have found evidence that carotenes reduce the risk of some cancers. The evidence is particularly strong for lung cancer, even after taking smoking into account. Every study that examined the role of carotene-rich foods found a reduced risk of lung cancer with higher intake. Carrots, sweet potatoes, cantaloupe, broccoli, and

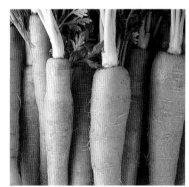
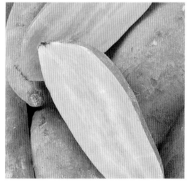
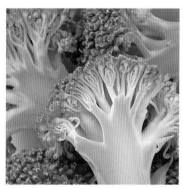

spinach are all particularly rich in carotenes.

- *Vitamin C:* Scientific studies have shown that this vitamin has a protective effect particularly for the esophagus, oral cavity, and stomach, as well as for cancers of the pancreas, rectum, and cervix. Citrus fruits and juices and green vegetables are rich in vitamin C.
- *Vitamin E:* In scientific studies vitamin E has been linked to reduced risks of oral, stomach, and other cancers. Nuts, seeds, some cereals, and vegetable oils are rich in vitamin E.
- *Lycopene:* It has been suggested that lycopene can protect against damage to cells and so reduce the risk of cancers particularly prostate, breast, colon, stomach, and lung cancer. Lycopene is classed as an antioxidant, which you can find in tomatoes and tomato products. Canned and pureed tomatoes are particularly good sources of lycopene.

In a recent scientific review of 19 studies, 16 showed an inverse association between cereal fiber intake and colon cancer, that is, a low intake of fiber from cereals is linked to the development of cancer of the colon. Only three studies failed to show a relationship. A consensus statement by 17 European cancer experts on the basis of the review concluded that, "a diet rich in high fiber cereal foods is associated with a reduced risk of colorectal cancer."

Not convinced of the benefits from wholegrain carbs, fruits, and vegetables? Well, the American Institute for Cancer Research most certainly is. Here are their guidelines for cancer prevention.

- Choose a diet rich in a variety of plant-based foods.
- Eat plenty of vegetables and fruits.
- Maintain a healthy weight and be physically active.
- Drink alcohol only in moderation.
- Select foods low in fat and salt.
- Prepare and store foods safely.
- Do not use tobacco in any form.

For more information check out their website ***www.aicr.org***

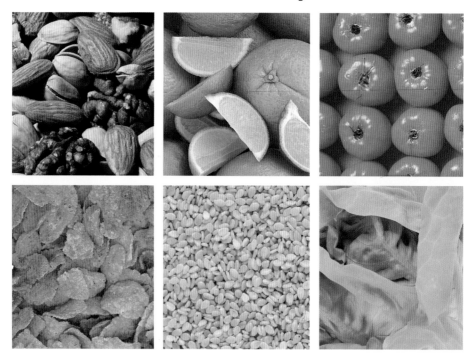

Recipes

Recipes

introduction

Planning and eating healthier meals can often be difficult and time consuming, especially if you are working and have a family to feed and look after. It is tempting to just pop to the grocery store and pick up a ready-to-cook meal or better still pick up the phone and dial for take-out without even having to move from your couch.

Now that you've resolved to eat healthier carbs, why not go a step further and take control of what goes into your body. Rather than trying to work out what ingredients have gone into making the pizza you've ordered or

the TV dinner in the back of your freezer, why not look go back to the basics and cook up some of the following recipes from scratch. That way, you can be in the driving seat and know exactly what you're eating and how many calories and how much fat you are consuming with each meal. Enjoy!

Please note: Where recipes specify salt and pepper to taste, these have not been added into the nutritional analysis. For reference, 1 tsp. salt contains approximately 2000mg sodium and 1 tsp. Losalt contains 655mg.

Soups

vegetable soup with quinoa

serves 4

Ingredients

1 tbsp. olive oil
1 garlic clove, crushed
2 large onions, chopped
4 oz. carrots, diced
2 oz. celery, diced
2 oz. green bell pepper, chopped
scant $1/2$ cup quinoa, rinsed
1 quart vegetable broth or water
2 bay leaves
salt and freshly ground black pepper
    to taste
handful of fresh flat-leaf parsley

Method

- Heat the oil in a large pan over a medium heat until hot. Add the garlic, onions, carrots, celery, green bell pepper, and quinoa. Sauté for about 5 minutes, stirring occasionally.
- Add the broth or water and bay leaves and bring to a boil.
- Reduce the heat to a simmer, cover, and cook for about 25–30 minutes, or until the quinoa is soft.
- Season to taste with salt and pepper.
- Sprinkle over with parsley just before serving.

Nutritional Analysis Per Serving

123cal, 3.7g protein, 3.8g fat,
19.8g carbohydrates, 10.5g sugars, 2.9g fiber,
28mg sodium

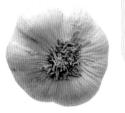

fava bean and squash chowder

serves 6

Ingredients

1 large onion, chopped
1 garlic clove, crushed
8 oz. butternut squash, diced
7 oz. fava beans, soaked overnight
1 1/2 pints vegetable broth
8 fl. oz. low-fat milk salt and freshly ground
   black pepper to taste
handful of cilantro leaves

Method

- Sweat the onion and garlic in a large pan over low heat for about 10–15 minutes or until the onions have softened and turned translucent.
- Add the butternut squash, fava beans, and vegetable broth. Bring the mixture to a boil, cover and simmer for about 1–1 1/2 hours or until the beans are soft.
- Transfer the soup to a blender and puree until smooth.
- Return the soup to the pan and add in the milk. Bring the soup back to a fast simmer and serve, garnished with cilantro leaves.

Nutritional Analysis Per Serving

102cal, 7.3g protein, 0.6g fat, 18.1g carbohydrates, 8.4g sugars, 4.4g fiber, 171mg sodium

leek and barley soup

serves 4

Ingredients

11 1/2 oz. leeks, sliced
1 large onion, chopped
1 3/4 oz. pearl barley
1 3/4 pints vegetable broth
salt and freshly ground black pepper to taste
1/4 cup sour cream, half-fat
handful of flat-leaf parsley

- Sweat the leeks and onion in a large pan over low heat for about 10–15 minutes or until the leeks have softened and the onions have turned translucent.
- Add the pearl barley and vegetable broth and bring to a boil. Cover and let simmer over a low heat for about 1 hour or until the pearl barley is soft.
- Season to taste. Divide soup between six bowls, garnish with a dollop of sour cream and flat-leaf parsley before serving.

Nutritional Analysis Per Serving

105cal, 3.4g protein, 2.6g fat, 18.1g carbohydrates, 5.5g sugars, 2.6g fiber, 8mg sodium

butternut squash soup

serves 4

Ingredients

1 large onion, peeled, coarsely chopped

5 oz. carrots, peeled, cut into large chunks

1 butternut squash (about 1^1/$_2$lb.), peeled and cut into large chunks

2^1/$_2$ cups vegetable broth

1 slice fresh gingerroot

8 oz. firm tofu (drained weight)

Method

• Sweat the onion in a large pan over low heat for about 10 minutes.

• Add the carrots, butternut squash, ginger, and broth. Increase the heat and bring to a boil.

• Reduce the heat to low and let simmer for about 25–30 minutes until all the vegetables are soft.

• Add the tofu, stir, and return the soup to a boil over medium heat.

• Transfer the mixture to a food processor or blender and process for about 30 seconds until the soup is smooth and creamy. Serve at once.

Nutritional Analysis Per Serving

145cal, 8.0g protein, 3.1g fat, 22.9g carbohydrate,
14.3g sugars, 4.5g fiber, 21mg sodium

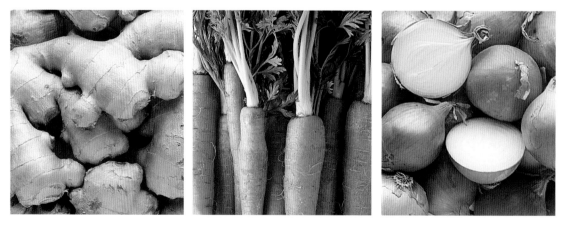

Light snacks and salads

lettuce wraps

serves 4

Ingredients

6 dried Chinese mushrooms
2 romaine lettuces
1 tbsp. rapeseed or olive oil
4 garlic cloves, crushed
2 large shallots, sliced
2 slices gingerroot, chopped
2 fresh red chilies, seeded, sliced
8 canned water chestnuts, diced
2 oz. canned bamboo shoots, diced
$5^1/2$oz. carrots, peeled and diced
1 heaping tbsp. hoisin sauce
2 tsp. shoyu or tamari sauce
freshly ground black pepper
14 oz. package silken firm tofu, diced
   (drained weight)
$1^1/2$ tsp. cornstarch
$^2/3$ cup vegetable broth
4 scallions, sliced
$^1/2$ cup toasted walnuts

Method

- To reconstitute the dried Chinese mushrooms, place them in a heatproof bowl, add enough water to cover, then place a plate over the top to keep the steam in. Set aside for 20–30 minutes. Drain, remove stalks, then squeeze the water out of the mushrooms, and coarsely chop.
- Separate the lettuce leaves, wash, pat dry, and set aside in the refrigerator.
- Heat the oil in a nonstick pan or preheated wok over high heat until piping hot, add the garlic, shallots, ginger, and chili and stir-fry for two minutes.
- Add in the water chestnuts, bamboo shoots, and carrots, stir-fry for about 5 minutes before stirring in the hoisin and shoyu or tamari sauces and black pepper. Next add the tofu and stir gently to mix, add the vegetable broth and bring to a boil.
- Meanwhile, in a small bowl, dissolve the cornstarch in a small amount of water (about 1 tbsp.) to make a paste. Push the ingredients to the sides of the wok and pour the cornstarch paste into the middle. When the sauce starts to thicken, stir in the rest of the mixture and mix well.
- Finally toss in the scallions and walnuts.
- To serve, take a piece of lettuce, spoon over some tofu vegetable mixture, and fold it up into a package before eating.

Nutritional Analysis Per Serving

123cal, 3.7g protein, 3.8g fat, 19.8g carbohydrates,
10.5g sugars, 2.9g fiber, 28mg sodium

watermelon salad

serves 4

Ingredients

1 bunch watercress
1lb. 5 oz. gold or red watermelon, chunks, seeds removed
10^1/$_2$oz. mozzarella cheese, sliced and cut into chunks
handful fresh basil leaves, coarsely torn
2 tbsp. sesame seeds

Raspberry vinaigrette dressing
1 shallot, chopped finely
2 tbsp. raspberry vinegar
1 tbsp. olive oil
Freshly ground black pepper

Method

- Mix the ingredients of the vinaigrette in a screw-top jar and set aside.
- Place the watercress leaves in the bottom of a large plate, arrange the watermelon and mozzarella cheese chunks over the top. Let chill until ready to serve.
- Just before serving, sprinkle the basil leaves and sesame seeds over the top and drizzle with the vinaigrette dressing.

Nutritional Analysis Per Serving

211cal, 9.5g protein, 14.5g fat,
11.0g carbohydrates, 11.0g sugars, 1.0g fiber,
163mg sodium

chickpea (garbanzo bean) salad

serves 4

Ingredients

2 garlic cloves, crushed
1 tbsp. extra virgin olive oil
2 tbsp. lime juice
2 shallots, finely chopped
3 tbsp. fresh chives, chopped
3 tbsp. fresh flat-leaf parsley, chopped
6 oz. canned chickpeas, drained
2 large red apples, unpeeled and chopped
salt and freshly ground black pepper to taste

Method

- Mix the garlic, olive oil, lime juice, shallots, and herbs in a serving dish. Add the chickpeas and apples. Season to taste and mix thoroughly before serving.

Nutritional Analysis Per Serving

144cal, 3.8g protein, 6.9g fat,
17.7g carbohydrates, 10.6g sugars, 3.6g fiber,
99mg sodium

fruity buckwheat salad

serves 6

Ingredients

9 oz. buckwheat groats, roasted
generous $2^1/2$ cups vegetable broth
$^1/4$ cup pumpkin seeds
generous $^1/3$ cup dried cranberries
$^1/2$ cucumber, diced

Dressing:
juice of 2 limes
zest from $^1/2$ lime
2 tbsp. extra virgin olive oil
1 tbsp. fresh dill
salt and freshly ground black pepper to taste

Method

- In a large saucepan, place the buckwheat and broth and bring to a boil. Cover the pan and simmer over low heat for approximately 30 minutes. All the broth should have been absorbed.
- Add the dressing ingredients to the warm buckwheat and then set aside to cool.
- When cool, mix in the pumpkin seeds, cranberries, and cucumber. Season to taste with salt and pepper.

Nutritional Analysis Per Serving

256cal, 5.8g protein, 8.2g fat, 42.6g carbohydrates,
6.2g sugars, 1.6g fiber, 4mg sodium

crunchy lentil salad

serves 4

Ingredients

scant $^7/8$ cup green lentils
4 cups vegetable broth
1 medium white onion, finely chopped
3 oz. carrots, finely chopped
1 large red apple, unpeeled diced
1 tbsp. fresh parsley, finely chopped
1 tbsp. olive oil
1 tbsp. balsamic vinegar
salt and pepper to taste
$5^1/2$oz. feta cheese
1 heaping tbsp. raisins

Method

- Place the lentils and broth in a saucepan, bring to a boil, cover, and let simmer for 30–35 minutes or until the lentils are cooked. Drain well and let cool.
- Mix lentils with the onion, carrots, apple, parsley, olive oil, and vinegar and season to taste.
- Mix in the feta cheese and raisins before serving. Serve with cold boiled new potatoes.

Nutritional Analysis Per Serving

214cal, 11.5g protein, 3.8g fat, 35.6g carbohydrates,
13.8g sugars, 5.7g fiber, 17mg sodium

107

fruity chicken salad with rice

serves 4

Ingredients

9 oz. cooked brown rice
12 dried apricots, chopped
$1/2$ cup toasted almonds
$1/2$ bulb fennel, sliced
1 tbsp. mango chutney
Juice 1 lime
4 cooked chicken breasts, diced
1 cucumber, diced
generous $1/2$ cup strained
   unflavored yogurt
2 tbsp. cilantro, chopped
Salt and freshly ground black pepper

Method

• Simply mix all of the ingredients in a large bowl and season to taste.

> **Nutritional Analysis Per Serving**
>
> 395cal, 28.5g protein, 16.3g fat,
> 36.4g carbohydrates, 16.0g sugars, 4.3g fiber,
> 166mg sodium

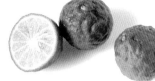

lime pasta salad with shrimp

serves 4

Ingredients

2 tbsp. olive oil
$1 1/2$ tbsp. lime juice
2 tbsp. tomato juice
1 tbsp. fresh dill, chopped
9 oz. cooked whole-wheat pasta
12 cherry tomatoes, halved
$4 1/2$ oz. black olives
7 oz. cooked shrimp, shelled
1 scallion, finely chopped
black pepper to taste

Method

• Combine olive oil, lime juice, tomato juice, and dill to make a dressing.
• Place pasta in a large bowl; add dressing, tomatoes, olives, shrimp, and scallion. Season with salt and pepper, mix to combine.

> **Nutritional Analysis Per Serving**
>
> 205cal, 14.6g protein, 10.7g fat,
> 13.5g carbohydrates, 2.1g sugars, 3.2g fiber,
> 2656mg sodium

shrimp and grapefruit salad

serves 4

Ingredients

14 oz. fresh shrimp, shelled and deveined
2 large grapefruits or 1 large pomelo,
 peeled, segmented
1 small red onion, sliced thinly
1 small ripe avocado, chopped
4 tbsp. lemon and fish sauce (see below)
1 tbsp. fresh cilantro leaves, chopped

Method

- Bring a pan of water to a boil, add the shrimp and cook until they are pink, this should take about 1–2 minutes. Remove with a slotted spoon and let cool.
- In a serving dish, place the grapefruit, onion, and avocado. Arrange the shrimp over the top and drizzle the lemon and fish sauce over this. Toss to mix well.
- Sprinkle the cilantro leaves over the top and serve at once.

Nutritional Analysis Per Serving

182cal, 19.7g protein, 5.7g fat, 14.0g carbohydrate,
13.2g sugars, 2.9g fiber, 432mg sodium

lemon and fish sauce

serves 4

Ingredients

2 fresh red chilies, seeded and chopped
1/2 garlic clove, crushed
2fl. oz. fresh lemon juice
2fl. oz. Thai fish sauce
3 tbsp. brown sugar
1/2 cup water

Method

- In a screwtop jar, mix all the ingredients together.
- This will keep in the refrigerator for a week. Serve with Shrimp and Grapefuit Salad, above, or other suitable shellfish dishes and salads.

Nutritional Analysis Per Serving

10cal, 0.2g protein, 0g fat, 2.5g carbohydrate,
2.0g sugars, 0g fiber, 235mg sodium

apple and fennel salad with tofu and chive dressing

serves 4

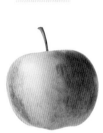

Ingredients

2 apples, preferably Fuji, cored, sliced
2 Asian pears (Chinese Nashi pears), cored, sliced
1 large Florence fennel bulb, thinly sliced
2 tbsp. toasted walnuts

Tofu and chive dressing:
3oz. silken tofu
1 tbsp. rice vinegar
1 tbsp. apple juice
$1/2$ garlic clove, crushed
2 tbsp. fresh chives, snipped

Method

- Blend all of the ingredients for the dressing together in a food processor or blender.
- Pour into a screw-top jar and place in the refrigerator until ready to use (it will keep for about one week in the refrigerator).
- Place the apples, pears, and fennel in a salad bowl, add the dressing, and toss until mixed.
- Sprinkle with walnuts just before serving.

Nutritional Analysis Per Serving

359cal, 9.8g protein, 22.7g fat,
30.1g carbohydrate, 28.2g sugar, 7.3g fiber,
24mg sodium

tabbouleh salad with chickpeas (garbanzo beans)

serves 6

Ingredients

$5^1/2$ oz. bulgur wheat
15fl. oz. (generous $1^3/4$ cups) vegetable broth
1 heaping tbsp. fresh flat-leaf parsley, chopped
1 heaping tbsp. fresh mint, chopped
4 vine-ripened medium tomatoes, diced
$1/2$ cucumber, diced
2 scallions, chopped
$2^1/2$oz. canned chickpeas
juice of 1 lime
2 tbsp. extra virgin olive oil
$1/2$ garlic clove, crushed
salt and freshly ground black pepper to taste

Method

- In a covered pan, bring the vegetable broth to a boil. Remove from the heat; add the bulgur wheat, stir, and cover. Let steam for about 30 minutes, or until all of the broth has been absorbed and the bulgur wheat has softened.
- Fluff up the bulgur wheat with a fork, add the remaining ingredients, and stir well to mix. Season to taste.
- Serve as a side salad at room temperature.

Nutritional Analysis Per Serving

148cal, 3.9g protein, 4.7g fat,
23.2g carbohydrates, 2.1g sugars, 1.2g fiber,
35mg sodium

spinach salad with rice and toasted almonds

serves 4

Ingredients

9oz. wild rice
1 red bell pepper, sliced thinly
2 tbsp. feta cheese
2 scallions, chopped
1 tbsp. fresh basil, chopped
1 tbsp. fresh chervil, chopped
2 tbsp. toasted almonds
7 oz. young leaf spinach

Dressing
$1/2$ white onion, minced
1 garlic clove, crushed
3 tbsp. lime juice
1 tbsp. extra virgin olive oil
$1/2$ tsp. Dijon mustard

Method

- Cook the wild rice according to the instructions on the package, drain and set aside to cool.
- In a serving bowl, mix the wild rice, red bell pepper, feta cheese, scallions, and herbs together. Add almonds.
- Whisk the dressing ingredients (garlic, onion, lemon juice, olive oil, and mustard) together in a separate bowl.
- Pour the dressing over the rice, nuts, and herbs mixture.
- Serve on a bed of washed young leaf spinach with toasted whole-wheat pita bread

Nutritional Analysis Per Serving

398cal, 17.3g protein, 13.3g fat, 54.5g carbohydrates,
6.1g sugars, 2.7g fiber, 484mg sodium

poor man's caviar

serves 6 as an appetizer

Ingredients

1 large eggplant
$1/2$ tbsp. extra virgin olive oil
2 shallots, finely chopped
1 garlic clove, crushed
7oz. low-fat cream cheese
generous $1/3$ cup vegetable broth
juice from 1 lime
salt and freshly ground black pepper to taste
pinch of cayenne pepper

Method

- Preheat an oven to 400F/200C.
- Place the eggplant on a foil-lined roasting pan and bake in the middle of the oven for 30–35 minutes until it is soft and wrinkly. Let cool before chopping it up into large chunks.
- Heat the oil in a sauté pan and then add in the shallots and garlic. Reduce the heat to low and sweat the shallots for about 10 minutes or until soft. Let cool.
- Place the eggplant, shallots, garlic, and cream cheese in a blender, add the broth and lime juice, and blend until smooth.
- Season to taste with salt and pepper.
- Serve the "caviar" in a large dish, garnished with a pinch of cayenne pepper.

Nutritional Analysis Per Serving

123cal, 3.7g protein, 3.8g fat,
19.8g carbohydrates, 10.5g sugars,
2.9g fiber, 28mg sodium

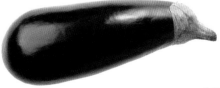

Main dishes

red thai curry with tofu and mixed vegetables

serves 4

Ingredients

1 tbsp. rapeseed or olive oil
2 tbsp. red curry paste
1–2 fresh green chilies, seeded and sliced
scant 1 cup light coconut milk
1 cup vegetable broth
1lb. eggplant, diced
12 baby corn
4 oz. snow peas
4 oz. carrots, peeled and sliced
4 oz. fresh shiitake mushrooms, halved
1 large green bell pepper, sliced
4½oz. canned sliced bamboo shoots, drained
1 tbsp. Thai fish sauce
1 tbsp. honey
2 kaffir lime leaves
14 oz. firm tofu, (drained weight) cut into 2 in. cubes
1 large handful of Thai basil leaves
1 handful of toasted cashews

Method

- Heat the oil in a skillet, fry the red curry paste and chilies for 1 minute, then stir in half of the coconut milk (from the thickened part, which is at the top of the can), cook while stirring constantly for 2 minutes.
- Add the vegetable broth and bring to a boil. Toss in the eggplant, return the mixture to a boil, and let simmer for about 5 minutes. Add the remaining vegetables and cook for an additional 5–10 minutes.
- Stir in the fish sauce, honey, remaining coconut milk, and lime leaves, then let simmer for an additional 5 minutes stirring occasionally. Add the tofu cubes and mix well.
- Top with torn Thai basil leaves and toasted cashews before serving.

Nutritional Analysis Per Serving

254cal, 13.3g protein, 13.8g carbohydrate, 11.0g sugars, 16.3g fat, 4.8g fiber, 482mg sodium

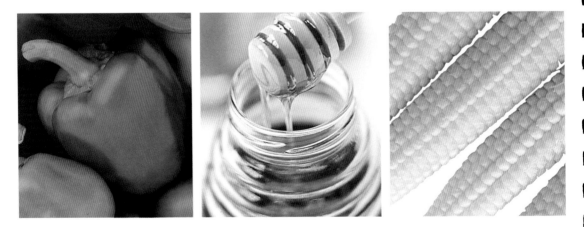

polenta with szechwan relish

serves 4

Ingredients

Polenta:
9³/₄oz. (scant 1⁷/₈ cups) coarse grain yellow cornmeal
scant 7⁵/₈ cups or 1.9 quarts vegetable broth

Relish:
8 oz. fresh tomatoes, diced
4 oz. cucumber, diced
1 fresh red chili, seeded and sliced
2 tbsp. scallions, thinly sliced
¹/₄ garlic clove, crushed
¹/₄ tsp. brown sugar
1 tbsp. lime juice
2 tbsp. fresh cilantro leaves, chopped
¹/₄ tsp. freshly ground black pepper

Method

- To prepare the polenta, bring the stock to a boil in a large pan. Increase the heat to medium.
- Place the cornmeal in a pitcher, and pour the cornmeal into the hot stock in a constant stream, stirring with a wooden spoon all the time. Cook the cornmeal for about 40–45 minutes, stirring constantly. Pour this into a square plastic container that has been rinsed out with cold water and flatten the top with a rubber spatula. Cover and let chill in the refrigerator until cold.
- Meanwhile, prepare the relish by mixing all the ingredients in a bowl.
- Turn the cornmeal out on a cutting board and cut into thick, square slices or whatever shapes you like. Brown the slices in a nonstick skillet and serve with the relish on the side.

Nutritional Analysis Per Serving

270cal, 7.2g protein, 2.5g fat, 53.4g carbohydrates,
3.0g sugars, 2.3g fiber, 8mg sodium

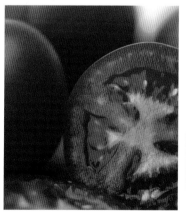
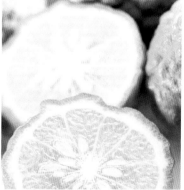
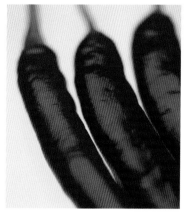

millet, bell pepper, and fennel au gratin

serves 4

Ingredients

10¹/₂oz. millet
¹/₂ tbsp. olive oil
1 large onion, chopped
1 garlic clove, crushed
1 large red bell pepper, chopped
1 large green bell pepper, chopped
7 oz. fennel, sliced
generous 1³/₄ cup tomato juice
1 tbsp. tomato paste
2 bay leaves
handful of fresh thyme
salt and freshly ground black pepper
3¹/₂oz. mature half-fat cheddar
  cheese, grated

Method

- Preheat the oven to 375F/190C.
- Bring a large pan of water to a boil. Stir in the millet and bring the mixture to a boil. Cover and let simmer for about 15–20 minutes or until soft. Drain and set aside.
- In a sauté pan, heat the oil until hot; add in the onion and garlic, and stir-fry for about 1 minute, or until brown.
- Add the two peppers and fennel and stir-fry for two minutes.
- Add the tomato juice, tomato paste, millet, bay leaves, and thyme, season to taste. Stir to mix and then pour into an ovenproof dish.
- Bake in the middle of the oven for 45 minutes, sprinkle over the cheese, and bake for an additional 30 minutes before serving.

Nutritional Analysis Per Serving

433cal, 19.0g protein, 9.2g fat, 65.8g carbohydrates,
9.6g sugars, 3.7g fiber, 426mg sodium

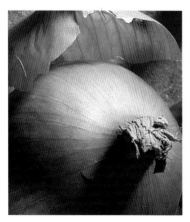
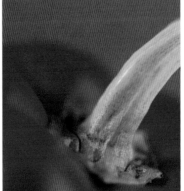
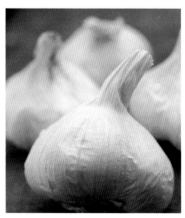

spinach and ricotta quiche

makes one 8in. quiche

Ingredients

4^1/$_2$oz. whole-wheat flour
1^3/$_4$oz. low-fat spread
1–2 tbsp. cold water
12 oz. ricotta cheese
7 oz. cooked spinach
scant 1 cup low-fat milk
2 medium eggs
nutmeg, salt, and white pepper, to taste

Method

• Preheat the oven to 400F/200C.
• Sift the flour into a bowl. Rub in the low-fat spread and add enough water to bind. Roll out on a lightly floured counter and use to line an 8in. tart pan.
• Bake the pastry shell blind for 10–12 minutes. Reduce the heat to 180C/350F.
• Place the ricotta cheese and spinach in the base of the pastry shell.
• Whisk the milk and eggs together and season to taste with nutmeg, pepper, and salt.
• Pour into the pastry shell and place on a baking sheet in the preheated oven for 30–40 minutes or until the filling has set.
• Serve this with sliced beefsteak tomatoes.

Nutritional Analysis Per Serving

329cal, 19.3g protein, 17.1g fat,
26.1g carbohydrates, 5.0g sugars,
3.0g fiber, 278mg sodium

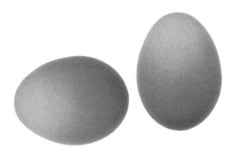

potato and mushroom frittata

serves 2

Ingredients

1 tbsp. olive oil
1 medium onion, sliced finely
6^1/$_4$oz. potatoes, unpeeled, sliced finely
5^1/$_2$oz. mushrooms, sliced
3 large eggs, whisked slightly
2 tbsp. chopped fresh parsley
Salt and pepper to taste

Method

• Heat oil in a non-stick skillet. Add onion, potatoes, and mushrooms and cook for a few minutes until brown, then reduce the heat down to low and cook, covered, for 20 minutes, or until the mixture has softened, stirring occasionally.
• Add eggs, parsley, add seasoning, stirring well to combine.
• Cook over low heat for 15–20 minutes, or until eggs are nearly set.
• Transfer the pan to a hot broiler and cook until top is set.
• Serve cold with cucumber and sliced tomatoes.

Nutritional Analysis Per Serving

351cal, 17.0g protein, 17.1g fat, 34.5g carbohydrates, 5.3g
sugars, 3.6g fiber, 154mg sodium

mixed bean bourguignonne

serves 4

Ingredients

1 tbsp. olive oil
1 large onion, chopped
3 garlic cloves, crushed
1 large carrot, chopped
1 large potato, chopped
2 tbsp. tomato paste
2 bay leaves
1 tbsp. fresh rosemary, chopped
1 1/2 cups red wine
1 quart vegetable broth
1lb. 2oz. cooked, mixed beans (for example, pinto, red kidney, fava beans)
8oz. mushrooms
salt and freshly ground black pepper to taste
3 tbsp. soured cream
handful of fresh flat-leaf parsley, chopped

Method

- Heat the oil in a large pan until hot; add the onions and sauté over medium heat until soft, about 5–7 minutes. Add the garlic, carrots, and potatoes and sauté for about 5 minutes.
- Add the tomato paste, bay leaves, rosemary, red wine, and vegetable broth and bring to a boil.
- Reduce the heat, cover, and let simmer for about 20–25 minutes or until the potatoes and carrots are cooked.
- Add the beans and mushrooms, and season to taste. Simmer for about 10 minutes or until the beans have warmed through.
- Trickle over with sour cream and sprinkle with parsley before serving.

Nutritional Analysis Per Serving

360cal, 15.8g protein, 10.2g fat, 39.1g carbohydrates,
10.9g sugars, 10.74 fiber, 333mg sodium

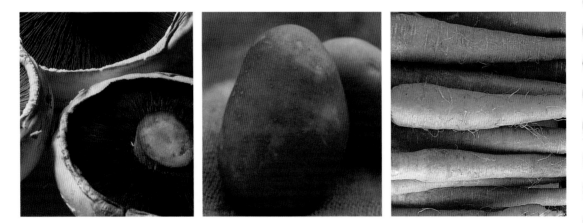

ratatouille

serves 4

Ingredients

2 tbsp. olive oil
1 tsp. cumin seeds
1 tbsp. cilantro seeds
1 large onion, chopped
3 garlic cloves, crushed
zest of $1/2$ lime
1 red bell pepper, chopped
1 green bell pepper, chopped
1lb. zucchini, diced
1lb. eggplant, diced
4 medium tomatoes, chopped
$51/2$oz. white mushrooms
8 oz. canned navy beans, drained
salt and freshly ground black pepper to taste
2 heaping tbsp. fresh flat-leaf parsley, chopped
large handful of fresh basil leaves, roughly torn

Method

• Heat the oil in a lidded pan over medium heat, add the cumin and cilantro seeds, and stir-fry for a few seconds. Add the onions and garlic, mix and fry for a few more seconds before tossing in the lime zest, bell peppers, zucchini, and eggplant. Stir to mix. Cover and let simmer over low heat for about 30 minutes, stirring occasionally.
• Add in the tomatoes and mushrooms and cook for an additional 30 minutes.
• Stir in the navy beans and season to taste with salt and pepper.
• Sprinkle with parsley and basil leaves before serving.
• Goes well with baked yam or warm corn tortillas.

Nutritional Analysis Per Serving

123cal, 3.7g protein, 3.8g fat, 19.8g carbohydrates,
10.5g sugars, 2.9g fiber, 28mg sodium

mixed bell pepper omelet

serves 2

Ingredients

2 tsp. olive oil
1 small red or orange bell pepper, diced ($1/4$in.)
1 small green bell pepper, diced ($1/4$in.)
2 tsp. red onion, diced ($1/4$in.)
4 egg whites, beaten
2 tsp. Parmesan cheese, freshly grated
2 tsp. snipped fresh chives

Method

• In a large nonstick skillet, heat the oil over medium heat.
• Add the bell peppers and red onion and sauté for about 5 minutes.
• Add the egg whites to the onion and bell pepper mixture and cook for a minute over medium-high heat, swirling the skillet to coat it evenly.
• Cook for about 30 seconds or until the eggs have set.
• Losen edges with a spatula before flipping the omelet over. Cook for an additional 45 seconds to 1 minute depending on how you like your omelet done.
• Sprinkle over with Parmesan cheese and chives before serving.

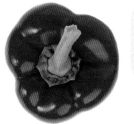

Nutritional Analysis Per Serving

78cal, 752g protein, 4.4g fat, 4.8g carbohydrates,
4.3 sugars, 1.5g fiber, 93mg sodium

soy loaf

serves 4

Ingredients

1 tbsp. olive oil
1 large onion, peeled and chopped
2 garlic cloves, crushed
2 celery stalks, chopped
1 large carrot, chopped
2 tomatoes, chopped
2 tbsp. tomato paste
9oz. canned soy beans, drained,
    mashed
4^{1}/$_{2}$oz. whole-wheat bread crumbs
handful chopped fresh parsley
1 tsp. dried oregano
1 medium egg
salt and freshly ground black pepper

Method

- Preheat the oven to 375F/190C.
- Heat the oil in a sauté pan, add the onion, garlic, celery, and carrot and fry over low-medium for about 15 minutes until the vegetables are tender.
- Add the tomatoes, tomato paste and cook for about 5 minutes.
- Stir in the mashed beans, bread crumbs, parsley, oregano, and egg. Season to taste with salt and pepper.
- Meanwhile, line a large loaf pan (1lb.) with waxed paper and grease with some oil. Pour the loaf mix into the pan and smooth down the top. Cover the top of the loaf with a piece of greased foil and bake in the center of the oven for about 1 hour.
- Turn the loaf out, take off foil, and peel off the waxed paper from the bottom before slicing and serving.
- Serve with applesauce.

Nutritional Analysis Per Serving

240cal, 15.9g protein, 7.5g fat, 29.1g carbohydrates,
11.0g sugars, 8.3g fiber, 246mg sodium

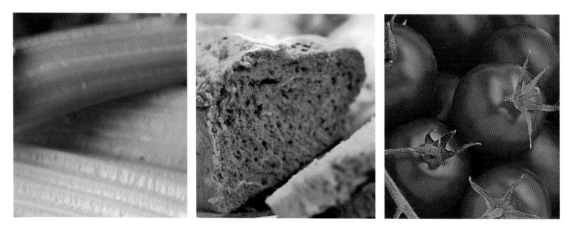

lentils with lemon grass and lime leaves

serves 4

Ingredients

$1/2$ tbsp. rapeseed or olive oil
$1/2$ tbsp. sesame oil
4 shallots, finely sliced
2 garlic cloves, crushed
2 fresh red chilies, seeded and sliced
15oz. dried brown/Puy lentils or yellow
    mung dal, washed and rinsed
3–4 cups vegetable broth
2 dried kaffir lime leaves
2 lemon grass stalks, cut into 1in. long pieces
    and crushed slightly
1 tsp. lemon zest
2 tbsp. shoyu or tamari sauce
large handful of Thai basil leaves

Method

• Heat the two oils over high heat in a pan until hot; add the shallots, garlic, and chilies and sauté for two minutes.
• Add the lentils and vegetable broth and bring to a boil.
• Stir in the lime leaves, lemon grass, lemon zest, and shoyu or tamari sauce. Reduce the heat and let simmer for about 25–30 minutes, stirring occasionally to prevent the lentils sticking to the bottom of the pan. Depending on which lentils you use, you may need to add more broth to ensure that they do not dry out.
• Stir in the torn basil leaves before serving.

Nutritional Analysis Per Serving

384cal, 32.8g protein, 56.8g carbohydrate, 2.7g sugars,
4.4g fat, 0.5g fiber, 267mg sodium

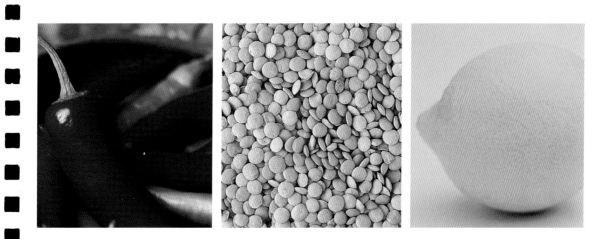

buckwheat or soba noodles with cashew and cilantro

serves 4

Ingredients

13oz. buckwheat or soba noodles
$1/2$ tbsp. rapeseed or olive oil
$1/2$ tsp. sesame oil
1 large onion, thinly sliced
4 garlic cloves, crushed
1 large carrot, thinly sliced
1 slice fresh ginger root, finely
  chopped
1 fresh red chili, seeded and sliced
4 tbsp. tamarind paste
scant $8^1/2$ cups vegetable broth
3 tbsp. shoyu or tamari sauce
$5^1/2$oz. cashews, unsalted, roasted
handful of fresh cilantro leaves,
  chopped

Method

- Bring a large pan of water to a boil. Once it is boiling, add the buckwheat or soba noodles, cover, and turn the heat off. Let the noodles steam for 5–7 minutes until slightly soft. Drain the noodles in a strainer and set aside.
- Meanwhile, heat the two different oils in a large pan over medium to high heat and add the onions, garlic, carrot, gingerroot, and chili. Cook for about 2–3 minutes stirring occasionally.
- Add the broth and tamarind paste and bring to a boil, reduce the heat, and let simmer for about 10 minutes before adding the shoyu or tamari sauce.
- To serve, divide the buckwheat noodles between 4–6 bowls and spoon the broth over the top.
- Sprinkle over the cashews and cilantro leaves just before serving.

Nutritional Analysis Per Serving

607cal, 20.8g protein, 90.4g carbohydrate, 19.9g sugar, 20.8g fat, 2.4g fiber, 1068mg sodium

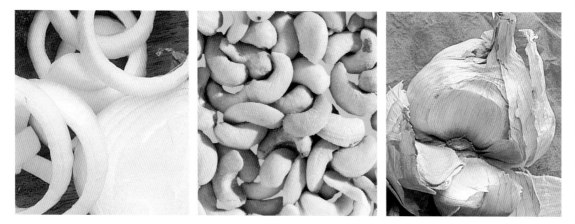

bean bake

serves 4

Ingredients

2 tbsp. olive oil
1 garlic clove crushed
2 large onions, finely chopped
1 green bell pepper, sliced
1 carrot, diced
1 tbsp. molasses
1 tbsp. low sodium soy sauce
1 tbsp. fresh thyme, chopped
1lb. 12oz. canned tomatoes
1lb. fava beans, canned
freshly ground black pepper
rock salt to taste
1^1/$_2$oz. Cheddar or Provolone cheese, crumbled
3 tbsp. fresh parsley, chopped
6oz. oatmeal

Method

- Heat 1 tbsp. olive oil in a pan; gently fry the garlic and onions until they are translucent. Increase the heat, add the green bell peppers, carrots, and stir-fry for two minutes, add the molasses, soy sauce, thyme, and canned tomatoes and cook for about 5 minutes over medium heat. Gently stir in the fava beans, then season to taste with pepper and rock salt.
- Spoon the mixture into a large greased ovenproof dish.
- Mix the cheese together with the parsley and oatmeal and sprinkle this mixture over the top of the bean mixture. Drizzle the remaining olive oil over the top.
- Cover the dish with foil and bake in a preheated oven 350F/180C for about 30 minutes. Remove the foil and cool for an additional 10 minutes, or until the top in golden brown.

Nutritional Analysis Per Serving

479cal, 21.9g protein, 14.8g fat, 69.0g carbohydrates,
19.4g sugars, 13.5g fiber, 767mg sodium

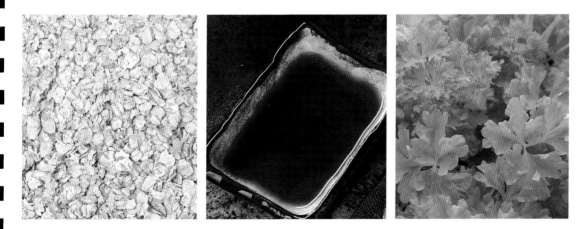

lentil and Roquefort lasagna

serves 6

Ingredients

generous 1 cup split red lentils
2 tbsp. olive oil
1 garlic clove, crushed
1 large onion, chopped
1lb. 12oz. canned tomatoes
1 tbsp. fresh rosemary
freshly ground black pepper
celery salt
1 tbsp. low-fat spread (suitable for cooking)
2 tbsp. whole-wheat flour
10 fl. oz. low-fat milk
8 oz. Roquefort cheese, crumbled
8 oz. whole-wheat lasagne sheets
1 tbsp. fresh parsley

Method

- Preheat the oven to 350F/180C.
- Cook the lentils in a pan of boiling water for about 35 minutes or according to the package instructions, until tender, and drain.
- Heat the oil in a sauté pan, add the garlic and onions, and cook over low heat until translucent. Add the canned tomatoes, rosemary, and cooked lentils to the pan, stir and bring to a boil. Season to taste with black pepper and celery salt, reduce the heat, cover, and let simmer for about 5 minutes. Remove from the heat.
- Make a white sauce using the low-fat spread, flour, and milk. Stir in the crumbled Roquefort.
- Layer the lentil mixture, lasagna sheets, and then the white sauce until it is all used up. Bake the lasagna for about 40 minutes, or until the top of the lasagna is golden brown. Sprinkle over with fresh parsley just before serving.

Nutritional Analysis Per Serving

534cal, 27.5g protein, 19.8g fat, 65.8g carbohydrates,
10.4g sugars, 7.4g fiber, 545mg sodium

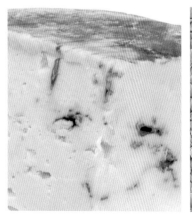
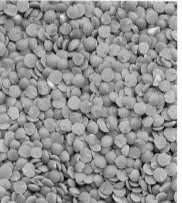
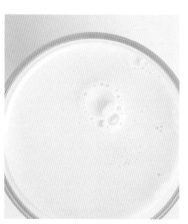

spiced beef and vegetable stew

serves 4

Ingredients

1 tbsp. rapeseed or olive oil
1 large onion, chopped
2 garlic cloves, crushed
4 slices fresh gingerroot
2 fresh chilies, seeded and sliced
1lb. lean round steak, cubed
$2^1/2$ cups beef broth
5 whole star anise
1 tsp. five spice powder
1 cinnamon stick
1 tsp. fennel seeds
2 dried kaffir lime leaves
1 lemon grass stalk, chopped
1 tsp. whole black peppercorns
2 tbsp. shoyu or tamari sauce
14 oz. carrots, cut into $^1/2$in. thick slices
1lb. mooli or turnips, cut into $^1/2$in. thick slices
1 tbsp. fresh chives, chopped

Method

• Heat the oil in a nonstick sauté pan or preheated wok over high heat until hot.
• Add the onion, garlic, gingerroot, and chilies, stir, and cook over medium heat for about 5–7 minutes.
• Increase the heat to high, add the beef, and fry for about 5–10 minutes until lightly browned, stirring occasionally.
• Add the broth, star anise, five spice powder, cinnamon stick, fennel seeds, lime leaves, lemon grass stalk, peppercorns, and shoyu. Mix and return the mixture to a boil before reducing the heat to simmer. Cover and cook over low heat for $1^1/2$ hours stirring occasionally.
• Add the carrots and mooli and continue cooking with the lid on for an additional 45 minutes, or until the vegetables have softened.
• To serve, skim any fat off the surface and sprinkle over with chopped chives.
• Goes well with boiled new potatoes.

Nutritional Analysis Per Serving

283cal, 30.5g protein, 10.7g fat, 17.8g carbohydrate,
14.6g sugars, 3.4g fiber, 393mg sodium

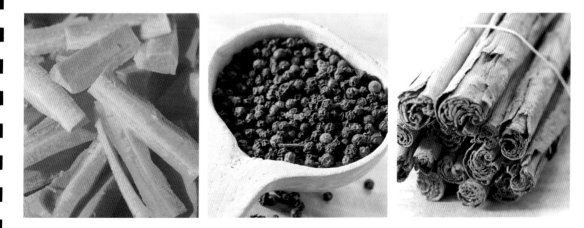

Side vegetables

parsnip and apple mash

serves 4

Ingredients

2lb. parsnips, peeled and chopped
   coarsely
1lb. Granny Smith apples, peeled,
   cored, chopped coarsely
$1/2$ cup half fat sour cream
freshly ground nutmeg
freshly ground black pepper to taste
handful toasted pine kernels
handful of snipped fresh chives

Method

- Place the parsnips in a large pan of water and bring to a boil. Cover, reduce the heat to a simmer and cook until soft, about 20–30 minutes. Drain and transfer to a blender.
- Meanwhile, place the apples in a small lidded pan. Add two tablespoons of water, and simmer with the lid on over low heat for about 10–12 minutes until soft. Place in the blender with the parsnips.
- Pour in the sour cream and process until smooth.
- Add the nutmeg, black pepper, and process for a second before placing the mash in a serving bowl.
- Sprinkle over with pine kernels and chives just before serving.

Nutritional Analysis Per Serving

291cal, 5.8g protein, 13.4g fat, 39.8g carbohydrates,
24.0g sugars, 11.9g fiber, 24mg sodium

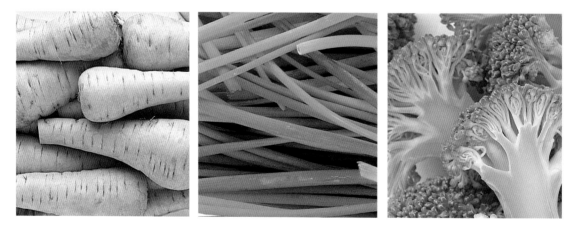

chili kale

serves 4 as a side dish

Ingredients

1 tbsp. olive oil
1 garlic clove, crushed
1 large white onion, chopped
2lb. 4oz. curly kale, chopped (stems removed)
2 tsp. lime juice
1 fresh red chili, seeded and chopped
1 tsp. Gomasio (Japanese ingredient—ground sesame seeds with small amount of salt)
1/2 tsp. freshly ground black pepper

Method

- Heat the oil in a pan and add the garlic and onion. Sauté for about 10 minutes, or until onion is translucent.
- Add the kale to the pan and stir-fry for about 5 minutes.
- Stir in the lime juice and red chili, season with Gomasio and pepper to taste and serve at once.
- Best served with a casserole.

Nutritional Analysis Per Serving

98cal, 9.1g protein, 4.1g fat, 6.8g carbohydrate,
5.4g sugars, 8.3g fiber, 150mg sodium

sesame broccoli

serves 4 as a side dish

Ingredients

1lb. broccoli florets
1 tbsp. toasted sesame seeds

Dressing
1 tsp. sesame oil
1 tbsp. shoyu or tamari sauce
1 garlic clove, crushed

Method

- Blanch the broccoli florets in boiling water for two minutes, drain, and place in a serving dish.
- Make a dressing out of sesame oil, shoyu or tamari sauce, and crushed garlic. Pour over broccoli florets.
- Just before serving, sprinkle the sesame seeds over the top.

Nutritional Analysis Per Serving

69cal, 6.3g protein, 3.6g fat, 2.7g carbohydrate,
1.9g sugars, 3.6g fiber, 136mg sodium

Breads

quinoa corn bread

makes 1 loaf (about 8 slices)

Ingredients

1 tbsp oil
$1/2$ cup cornmeal
scant 1 cup quinoa meal
$1/2$ tsp. baking soda
$1^1/2$ tsp. baking powder
1 tbsp. brown sugar
1 medium egg, lightly beaten
$2^1/2$ cups buttermilk

Method

- Preheat the oven to 425F/220C.
- If you can't get quinoa meal, first process quinoa grains in a blender or food processor.
- Oil a 9 x 9in. square pan with some oil.
- Place the cornmeal, quinoa meal, baking soda, baking powder, and sugar in a mixing bowl.
- Mix together the egg and buttermilk and add to the dry ingredients. Mix thoroughly together.
- Pour the mixture into the oiled pan and place in the center of the oven.
- Bake for about 25 minutes, or until the bread is golden brown.

Nutritional Analysis Per Serving

123cal, 7.2g protein, 2.7g fat, 32.2g carbohydrates,
5.2g sugars, 2.7g fiber, 205mg sodium

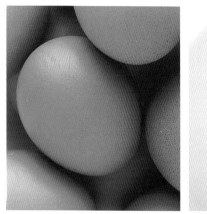

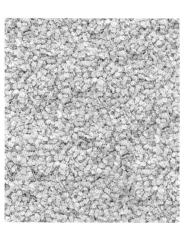

wild about rice bread

makes 1 loaf (about 8 slices)

Ingredients

2$^1/_2$ cups water
3 oz. wild rice
2 tbsp. brown sugar
2 tbsp. sunflower-seed oil
1 large egg
generous 1$^1/_5$ cups whole-wheat flour
2 tsp. baking powder
$^1/_2$ tsp. salt
$^1/_4$ cup pecans, chopped
$^1/_8$ cup sunflower seeds

Method

- Bring the water to a boil in a large pan, add the wild rice, and return to a boil. Cover and let simmer over low heat for about 45 minutes, or until the rice has absorbed all the water.
- Stir in the sugar and let cool.
- Meanwhile preheat the oven to 325F/160C. Line a large loaf pan with waxed paper and lightly oil.
- Add the oil and egg to the cooled rice mixture.
- Fold in the flour, baking powder, salt, pecans, and sunflower seeds.
- Pour the mixture into the loaf pan and bake in the center of the oven for 50–60 minutes or until cooked. If you insert a metal skewer into the center of the pan, it should come out clean. Let stand in the pan for about 10 minutes before turning it out and serving warm.

Nutritional Analysis Per Serving

211cal, 6.8g protein, 7.9g fat, 29.9g carbohydrates,
4.6g sugars, 2.9g fiber, 255mg sodium

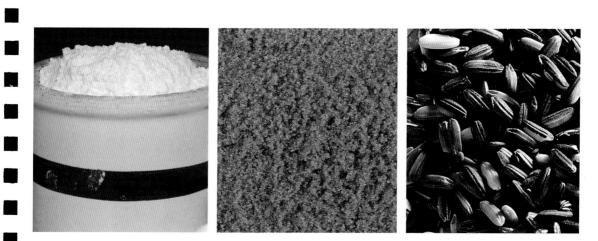

semolina bread

makes 2 loaves or around 16 slices

Ingredients

1/2 cup warm water
1/2 oz. active dry yeast
1/4 cup honey
1/4 cup olive oil
1 3/4 cups skim milk
generous 3/4 cup whole-wheat flour
scant 2 1/2 cups strong white bread
   flour
2 medium eggs
1lb. semolina
1 tbsp. poppy seeds

Method

- Place the warm water in a small bowl, sprinkle over the yeast, and set aside for about 7–10 minutes until the yeast starts to bubble.
- Mix the honey, oil, and milk in a small pan and heat until warm.
- Place the honey mixture into a blender or food processor and add in half of the white flour. Process until mixed well. With the machine running, gradually pour in the eggs and the yeast mixture until incorporated into the flour.
- Gradually blend in the rest of the flour (white and whole-wheat) and the semolina until a stiff dough is formed.
- Turn the dough onto a floured counter and knead well for about 10 minutes until smooth and shiny. Add more flour if you need to.
- Place the dough into an oiled bowl, turning it round so that it is coated with oil. Cover with a damp dish towel and set aside in a warm place until the dough has doubled in size—about 1 1/2 hours.
- Knock the dough back by kneading it for about 2–3 minutes. Cover again with a dish towel and let the dough rest in a warm place for about 30 minutes.
- Preheat the oven to 375F/190C.
- Turn the dough onto a floured counter and knead for a minute or so. Divide it into two and form them into 2 loaf pans (9 x 5 x 3 in.). Cover and set aside in a warm place for 45 minutes to 1 hour or until the loaves have filled and risen above the pans. Sprinkle the loaves with poppy seeds and bake in the middle of the oven for about 35–40 minutes or until they are browned and sound hollow when the bottom of the loaves are tapped.
- Remove and let cool on a wire rack before eating.

Nutritional Analysis Per Serving

250cal, 8.7g protein, 5.6g fat, 45.0g carbohydrates,
3.2g sugars, 1.8g fiber, 28mg sodium

pumpkin and sunflower tea bread

makes 2 loaves or around 16 slices

Ingredients

7 oz. all purpose flour
generous $3/8$ cup whole-wheat flour
2 tsp. baking powder
1 tsp. baking soda
1 tsp. ground cinnamon
$1/4$ tsp. ground nutmeg
generous $1/3$ cup corn oil
$1/2$ cup low-fat cream cheese
generous $3/4$ cup firmly packed brown sugar
2 medium eggs
$4^1/2$ oz. canned pumpkin pie filling
4oz. soured cream
$1/2$ cup sunflower seeds

Method

- Preheat the oven to 350F/180C.
- Lightly oil the sides of two 9 x 5 x 3 in. loaf pans. Line the bottom of the pans with oiled waxed paper.
- Mix the two flours, baking powder, baking soda, cinnamon, and nutmeg together in mixing bowl.
- In a blender, process the cream cheese, sugar, and oil together. Gradually add in the eggs. Blend before adding in the pumpkin pie filling and the sour cream.
- Pour in the dry ingredients and sunflower seeds and blend until just combined.
- Divide the batter between the two loaf pans and bake in the middle of the oven for about 55–60 minutes until the breads are cooked. If a toothpick pushed into the center of the loaves comes out clean, then the breads are ready.
- Let the loaves rest in the pans for about 10–15 minutes before turning out and cooling on a wire rack.

Nutritional Analysis Per Serving

214cal, 5.0g protein, 12.3g fat, 23.0g carbohydrates,
10.3g sugars, 1.0g fiber, 173mg sodium

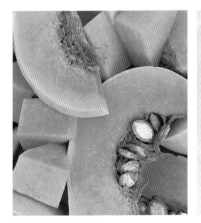

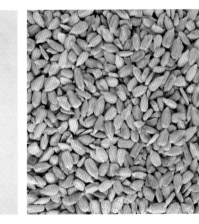

bran bread

makes 1 loaf (about 8 slices)

Ingredients

1lb. whole-wheat bread flour
$1/2$ tsp. salt
$1^1/2$ oz. All-Bran
1 tsp. active dry yeast
2 tbsp. sunflower-seed oil
$1^1/2$ cups warm milk
2 tbsp. warm water
2 tsp. sesame seeds

Method

- In a large mixing bowl, place the flour, salt, and All Bran cereal, add the yeast and oil, and mix in the warm milk and warm water.
- Turn the bread dough onto a floured counter and knead for about 10–15 minutes or until the dough is smooth and shiny. Mold it into whatever shape you like—round or cottage loaf or plait, and place onto a baking sheet that has been lined with oiled waxed paper.
- Cover the dough with a damp dish towel or lightly oiled plastic wrap and let stand in a warm place for about 1 hour, or until the dough has risen to double its original size.
- Meanwhile, preheat the oven to 425F/220C. Sprinkle with sesame seeds and bake in the center of the oven for about 30 minutes or until cooked. The bottom of the bread should sound hollow when tapped. Transfer to a wire rack to cool.

Nutritional Analysis Per Serving

241cal, 9.8g protein, 5.6g fat, 40.5g carbohydrates, 4.2g sugars, 6.4g fiber, 187mg sodium

Grains

bulgar wheat risotto with zucchini and porcini mushrooms

serves 4

Ingredients

1oz. dried porcini mushrooms
2 tbsp. olive oil
1 cinnamon stick (2 in. approx.)
1 large onion, chopped
1 garlic clove, crushed
10oz. zucchini, diced (1/2 in.)
3oz. coarse bulgur wheat
generous 3/4 cup vegetable broth
1 tbsp. fresh flat-leaf parsley, chopped

Method

- Place the dried porcini in a bowl, add enough water to cover, and let soak for about 2 hours. Lift the mushrooms out the liquid and squeeze out the juices.
- Heat the oil in a large pan over medium-high heat, add the cinnamon and cook for a few seconds before tossing in the onions and garlic. Sauté for 2 minutes.
- Add in the zucchini and bulgur wheat and stir for 3–4 minutes before adding in the vegetable broth and porcini mushrooms.
- Bring to a boil, cover, and let simmer for about 25 minutes over very low heat.
- Remove from the heat and set aside for 20 minutes keeping the lid on to allow the bulgur to steam to finish off cooking.
- Fluff up the grains and sprinkle over with parsley before serving.

Nutritional Analysis Per Serving

151cal, 5.0g protein, 6.0g fat, 18.5g carbohydrates,
4.9g sugars, 2.4g fiber, 74mg sodium

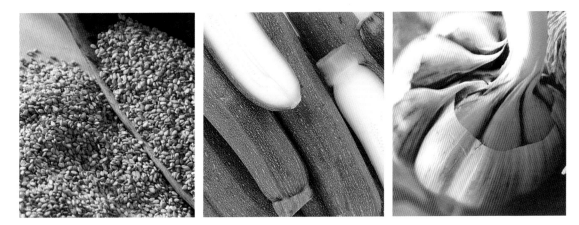

millet with chard and carrots

serves 4

Ingredients

1 tbsp. olive oil
1 large onion, chopped
2 carrots, diced
9 oz. millet grains
generous 1^3/$_4$ cups hot vegetable broth
2 fresh red chilies, seeded and finely chopped
1 bunch red chard leaves, chopped into strips
2 scallions, chopped finely
salt and freshly ground pepper to taste

Method

- Heat ^{1}/$_2$ tbsp. oil in a pan, add the onion and carrots and sauté over medium heat 2 minutes before adding the millet grains. Sauté for another 2 minutes before pouring in the hot vegetable broth. Bring to a boil, cover, and remove from the heat. Set aside to steam for about 1 hour.
- Heat the remaining ^{1}/$_2$ tbsp. oil in a sauté pan, add the chilies and sauté for a minute over medium heat.
- Toss in the chard leaves and sauté for a few minutes or until the chard wilts.
- Meanwhile, fluff up the millet grains and stir in the wilted leaves and chili mixture.
- Season to taste and sprinkle over with the scallions just before serving.

Nutritional Analysis Per Serving

285cal, 8.1g protein, 5.6g fat, 50.3g carbohydrates,
3.5g sugars, 1.0g fiber, 108mg sodium

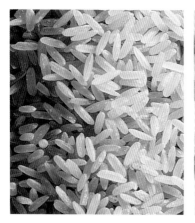
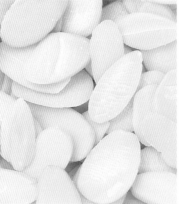
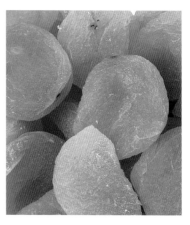

red rice

serves 4

Ingredients

4¹/₂oz. adzuki beans
5 cups water
1 cup brown rice
2 tbsp. black sesame seeds, toasted

Method

- Wash the adzuki beans and place them in a large pan. Cover with water and bring to a boil, then let simmer over low heat for about 45 minutes, or until they are tender. Set aside the liquid.
- Soak the brown rice in the reserved liquid for at least two hours and then drain.
- Mix the soaked brown rice and adzuki beans and place them in the top of a steamer. Steam over low heat for about 50–60 minutes, or until soft.
- Top with toasted sesame seeds before serving.
- Goes really well with a mixed green salad.

Nutritional Analysis Per Serving

322cal, 11.1g protein, 5.2g fat, 61.4g carbohydrates,
1.1g sugars, 5.0g fiber, 4mg sodium

mediterranean sweet couscous

serves 6

Ingredients

2 cups couscous
1 tbsp. orange blossom water
6 large dried apricots, cut into quarters
1 large handful of toasted almonds
1 large handful of toasted unsalted pistachio nuts
6 figs, cut into halves
scant 2¹/₂ cups strained unflavored yogurt

Method

- Place couscous in a large serving bowl, pour over enough hot water (about 2¹/₂ cups) to cover the top, add the orange blossom water, and cover with a plate or plastic wrap. Let stand for about 10 minutes, or until all the water has been absorbed. Fluff up the grains of couscous with a fork.
- Add the dried apricot and nuts, mix thoroughly, place halved figs over the top before serving with the strained unflavored yogurt.

Nutritional Analysis Per Serving

304cal, 9.8g protein, 10.8g fat, 46.0g carbohydrates,
20.2g sugars, 3.4g fiber, 74mg sodium

Fruity desserts

creamy tofu dessert with mixed berries

serves 4

Ingredients

1lb. 2oz. silken tofu
2 tbsp. lemon juice
1 tbsp. vanilla extract
4fl. oz. ($1/2$ cup) water
4fl. oz. ($1/2$ cup) pineapple juice
generous $3/4$ cup fresh strawberries
$1/2$ cup fresh raspberries
$1/2$ cup fresh blueberries
handful of fresh mint leaves

Method

- Place all the ingredients, except the berries, in a blender or food processor and whiz until smooth.
- Divide between four bowls and let chill until required.
- When ready to serve, top with mixed berries and mint leaves.

Nutritional Analysis Per Serving

130cal, 11.0g protein, 5.5g fat, 10.3g carbohydrates, 6.3g sugars, 1.0g fiber, 11mg sodium

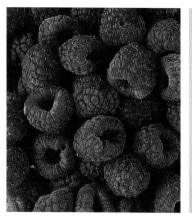
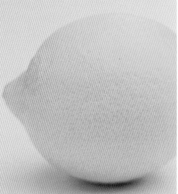
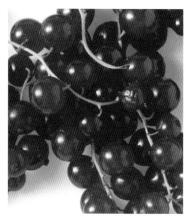

baked pears

serves 4

Ingredients

5 cups cranberry juice
1 cinnamon stick
$1/2$ vanilla bean
4 large ripe dessert pears, peeled
9 oz. strawberries
generous $1/2$ cup half-fat sour cream
1 tsp. rose water

- Heat the cranberry juice, cinnamon stick, and vanilla bean in a saucepan until the mixture is simmering.
- Add the pears and poach over low heat for about 15 minutes, carefully turning the pears once or twice during this time. Let the pears cool in the mixture.
- Remove the pears and place in a serving dish. Remove the cinnamon stick and vanilla bean from the liquid, and reduce the liquid by a half over a high heat.
- Meanwhile, de-husk the strawberries and cut into halves, then stir the strawberries into the sour cream and add the rose water.
- Serve the cooled pears with the rose flavored strawberry sour cream.

Nutritional Analysis Per Serving

310cal, 21.9g protein, 14.8g protein, 69.0g carbohydrates, 19.4g sugars, 13.5g fiber, 22mg sodium

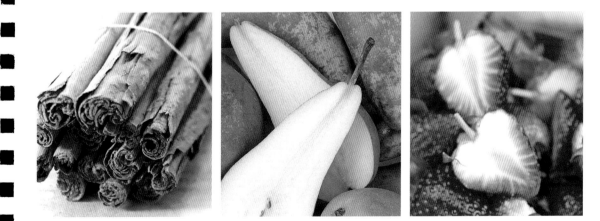

banana boats

serves 4

Ingredients

4 large bananas
4$^1/_2$oz. mascarpone or ricotta
cheese

Method

- Wrap the peeled bananas in foil. Bake in a preheated oven at 350F/180C for about 10–15 minutes. Unfold the foil and top with mascarpone cheese, serve in the foil packages.

Nutritional Analysis Per Serving

140cal, 4.1g protein, 3.7g fat, 23.8g carbohydrates, 21.5g sugars, 1.1g fiber, 32mg sodium

baked summer fruits

serves 4

Ingredients

generous 1 cup raspberries
4 peaches, halved and pitted
generous 1$^3/_4$ cups strawberries,
de-husked
generous $^5/_8$ cup black currants
9 oz. reduced fat unflavored yogurt
2 handfuls toasted pumpkin seeds

Method

- Mix the fruits together in a baking dish and bake in a preheated oven at 325F/160C for about 30 minutes.
- Divide into four tall glasses, top with two tablespoons of yogurt and a sprinkling of pumpkin seeds.

Nutritional Analysis Per Serving

158cal, 7.7g protein, 4.7g fat, 22.6g carbohydrates, 21.3g sugars, 5.4g fiber, 48mg sodium

stuffed baked apples

serves 4

Ingredients

4 cooking apples
1 cup whole-wheat bread crumbs
scant 3/8 cup chopped walnuts
1/3 cup golden raisins
1/2 tsp. ground cinnamon
grated rind from half a lemon

Method

- Preheat the oven to 350F/180C.
- Core the apples and set aside.
- Mix together the bread crumbs, walnuts, golden raisins, cinnamon, and lemon. Use this mixture to stuff the middle of the apples.
- Place the apples in a baking dish and bake in the middle of the oven for about 45–55 minutes.

Nutritional Analysis Per Serving

180cal, 3.6g protein, 9.1g fat, 22.5g carbohydrates, 17.5g sugars, 2.7g fiber, 65mg sodium

orange and date salad

serves 4

Ingredients

6 large oranges
6 large dried dates, chopped and pitted
scant 1 cup ruby grapefruit juice

Method

- Peel the oranges, cut into thick slices, and place in a large serving bowl. Add the chopped dates, mix, and pour over the grapefruit juice.
- Let the mixture infuse for at least 30 minutes in the refrigerator before serving.

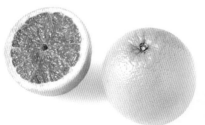

Nutritional Analysis Per Serving

145cal, 3.1g protein, 0.3g fat, 34.9g carbohydrates, 34.9g sugars, 4.2g fiber, 17mg sodium

Breakfast

bran muffins

Makes 24 mini muffins

Ingredients

$1/4$ cup corn oil
$1^5/8$ cup wheat bran cereal
$1^1/4$ cups low-fat milk
2 tbsp. whole-wheat flour
scant 1 cup all-purpose flour
scant $1/2$ cup firmly packed brown
   sugar
1 tbsp. baking powder
$1/2$ tsp. ground cinnamon
generous $1/2$ cup dried cranberries
pinch of salt
1 large egg

Method

- Preheat the oven to 400F/200C. Grease a 24-hole muffin pan with oil.
- In a large mixing bowl, combine the bran cereal and milk and set aside.
- In another bowl, mix together the dried ingredients. First sift the two types of flours together and then add in the sugar, baking powder, cinnamon, cranberries, and salt.
- Add the egg and oil to the softened cereal and milk mixture and mix thoroughly.
- Fold the dried ingredients into the egg, milk, and cereal mixture gently.
- Divide the batter between the muffin cups and bake in the center of the oven for about 20–25 minutes, or until done.
- Serve warm.

Nutritional Analysis Per Serving

82cal, 2.0g protein, 3.2g fat, 12.4g carbohydrates,
6.0g sugars, 0.5g fiber, 95mg sodium

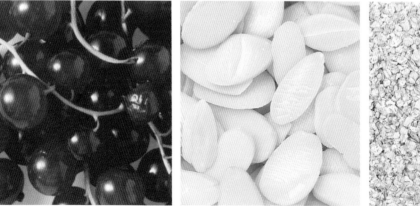

buckwheat pancakes

makes 12–14 pancakes

Ingredients

2^1/$_2$ cups warm skim milk
2^1/$_2$ tsp. active dry yeast
1 tsp. superfine sugar
2 tbsp. honey
generous ^{3}/$_4$ cup whole-wheat flour
generous ^{3}/$_4$ cup buckwheat flour
1 medium egg, beaten
1^1/$_2$ tbsp. corn oil

Method

- In a small bowl, place 5 tbsp. of warm milk and sprinkle in the yeast and superfine sugar. Stir and set aside in a warm place for about 7–10 minutes until the yeast starts to bubble.
- Place the whole-wheat and buckwheat flours in a mixing bowl. Make a well in the center of the flours and pour in the honey and yeast mixture. Stir and slowly add in the rest of the warm milk. Cover the bowl and set aside in a warm place for about 1 hour.
- Slowly add the beaten egg into the batter mixture, cover, and set aside again in a warm place for about 45 minutes.
- Heat a stovetop griddle pan over medium-high heat. Brush the bottom of the pan with oil. Pour the batter using a ladle to make a 4in. circle, repeat until the bottom of the pan is full.
- Cook the pancakes on each side for about a minute or so or until they are lightly browned.
- Remove the pancakes and keep warm.
- Continue making the pancakes in the same way.

Nutritional Analysis Per Serving

111cal, 5.0g protein, 2.7g fat, 18.0g carbohydrates,
5.1g sugars, 1.0g fiber, 32mg sodium

fruity oats

serves 4

Ingredients

2^1/$_2$ cups unsweetened orange juice
generous ^{1}/$_3$ cup water
pinch nutmeg
3 cups rolled oats
^{1}/$_2$ cup raisins
^{1}/$_2$ cup chopped toasted almonds
^{3}/$_8$ cup fresh blueberries
^{1}/$_2$ cup low-fat strained unflavored yogurt

Method

- Bring the juice, water, and cinnamon to a boil in a large pan.
- Add in the oats, raisins, and return to a boil.
- Reduce the heat to medium and cook for about 8–10 minutes, stirring occasionally until it reaches the consistency you want.
- Stir in the almonds and blueberries.
- Serve with yogurt.

Nutritional Analysis Per Serving

372cal, 10.4g protein, 6.0g fat, 73.9g carbohydrates, 28.3g
sugars, 5.3g fiber, 65mg sodium

birchermuesli

serves 4

Ingredients

3oz. rolled oats
generous 1 cup passion fruit juice
generous $2/3$ cup low fat strained
  plain yogurt
$1/3$ cup dried apricots
generous $1/8$ cup golden raisins
1 apple, peeled, grated
toasted walnuts
$4^1/2$oz. seedless grapes

Method

- Mix the oats and passion fruit juice together in a bowl and set aside for about 10 minutes.
- In another bowl, mix together the yogurt, dried apricots, golden raisins, and apple. Stir in the oats mixture.
- Cover and let chill in the refrigerator overnight.
- To serve, top with toasted walnuts and seedless grapes.
- Birchermuesli will keep in the refrigerator for up to three days.

Nutritional Analysis Per Serving

222cal, 6.7g protein, 5.7g fat, 38.6g carbohydrates,
26.3g sugars, 3.1g fiber, 42mg sodium

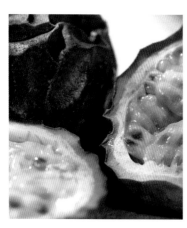
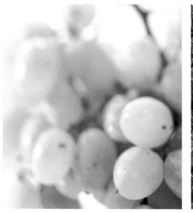
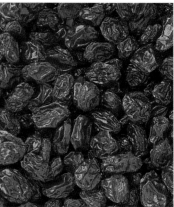

Nutrition Tables

Cereals

Food	Weight (grams)	Energy (cal)	Carbohydrate (grams)	Sugar (grams)	Fiber (grams)
All-Bran	100	264	75.9	19	32.3
All-Bran Bran Buds	100	276	79.9	27	39.9
Cheerios	100	365	76.2	5.5	11.9
Complete Oat Bran Flakes	100	350	77.0	20	13
Complete Wheat Bran Flakes	100	318	79.0	17	17.5
Corn grits, white, regular, quick, enriched, with water	100	60	13	not measured	0.2
Corn grits, yellow, regular, quick, enriched, with water	100	60	13	not measured	0.2
Crispy Wheaties 'n Raisins	100	348	80.6	40	6.2
Cream of rice, cooked with water	100	52	11.4	not measured	0.1
Crunchy Bran	100	333	84.2	not measured	17.8
Corn Grits,(Quaker), instant, butter flavor, water	100	69	14.2	not measured	0.9
Fiber One	100	205	80.0	2	47.5
Frosted Bran	100	338	84.7	32	11.2
Frosted Mini Wheats	100	340	81.4	20	10.7
Honey Graham Oh!s	100	414	84.2	45	2.6
Honey Nut Cheerios	100	383	80.9	38	5.2
Low-fat granola/raisins	100	367	79.4	29	6
Lucky Charms	100	387	83.9	43	4
Nutri-Grain Wheat	100	335	80	1	12.6
Original Shredded Wheat	100	340	81.5	1	11.5
Post Grape-Nuts, Flakes	100	365	77.3	18	8.8

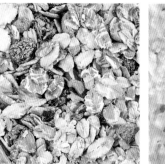 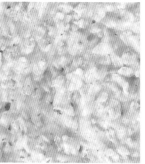 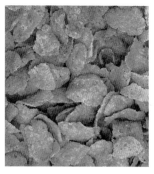

Grains

Food	Weight (grams)	Energy (cal)	Carbohydrate (grams)	Sugar (grams)	Fiber (grams)
Brown rice, boiled	100	141	32.1	1	0.8
Brown rice, raw	100	357	81.3	1	1.9
White rice, easy cook, boiled	100	138	30.9	Trace	0.1
White rice, polished, boiled	100	123	29.6	Trace	0.2
Noodles, egg, boiled	100	62	13	0	0.6
Noodles, plain, boiled	100	62	13	0	0.7
Macaroni, wholemeal, boiled	100	86	18.5	0	2.8
Macaroni, white, boiled	100	86	18.5	0	0.9
Spaghetti, wholemeal, boiled	100	113	23.2	1	3.5
Spaghetti, white, boiled	100	104	22.2	1	1.2
Brown bread, average	100	207	42.1	3	3.5
Granary bread	100	237	47.4	3	3.3
Naan bread	100	285	50.2	3	2
Pappadums, takeout	100	501	28.3	Trace	5.8
Paratha	100	322	43.2	1	4
Pita bread, white	100	255	55.1	3	2.4
Pumpernickel	100	219	45.8	2	7.5
Rye bread	100	219	45.8	2	4.4
Soda bread	100	258	54.6	3	2.1
Tortillas, made with wheat flour	100	262	59.7	1	2.4
White bread, French stick	100	263	56.1	3	2.4
White bread, high fiber	100	235	49.3	3	8.3
Wholemeal bread, average	100	217	42	3	5
Fruit cake, rich	100	343	59.9	49	1.5
Fruit cake, wholemeal	100	366	52.4	29	2.4
Gateau	100	337	43.4	32	0.4
Sponge cake	100	467	52.4	30	0.9

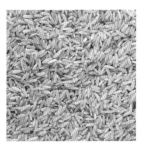
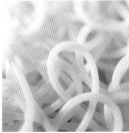
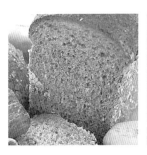
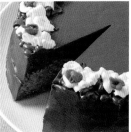

Nuts and Seeds

Food	Weight (grams)	Energy (cal)	Carbohydrate (grams)	Sugar (grams)	Fiber (grams)
Mixed nuts	100	607	7.9	4	6
Mixed nuts and raisins	100	481	31.5	29	4.5
Peanuts, dry roasted	100	589	10.3	4	6.4
Pecan nuts	100	689	5.8	4	4.7
Pine kernels	100	688	4	4	1.9
Pistachio nuts, roasted and salted	100	601	8.2	6	6.1
Pumpkin seeds	100	569	15.2	1	5.3
Sesame seeds	100	598	0.9	0	7.9
Sunflower seeds	100	581	18.6	2	6
Walnuts	100	688	3.3	3	3.5

Flour

Food	Weight (grams)	Energy (cal)	Carbohydrate (grams)	Sugar (grams)	Fiber (grams)
Chapati flour, brown	100	333	73.7	3	10.3
Chapati flour, white	100	335	77.6	2	4.1
Potato flour	100	328	75.6	3	5.7
Rye flour, whole	100	335	75.9	Trace	11.7
Soy flour, low fat	100	352	28.2	13	13.5
Wheat flour, white, plain	100	341	77.7	2	3.1
Wheat flour, wholemeal	100	310	63.9	2	9

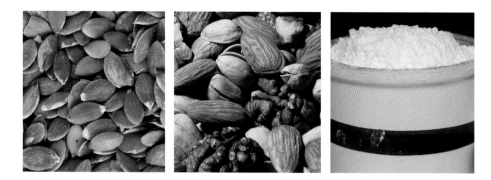

Beans

Food	Weight (grams)	Energy (cal)	Carbohydrate (grams)	Sugar (grams)	Fiber (grams)
Aduki beans, dried, boiled in unsalted water	100	123	22.5	1	5.5
Baked beans, canned in tomato sauce	100	81	15.1	6	3.5
Baked beans, canned in tomato sauce, reduced sugar, reduced salt	100	73	12.5	3	3.8
Blackeye beans, dried, boiled in unsalted water	100	116	19.9	1	3.5
Fava beans, canned, re-heated, drained	100	87	12.7	1	5.2
Fava beans, frozen, boiled in unsalted water	100	81	11.7	1	6.5
Lima beans, canned, re-heated, drained	100	77	13	1	4.6
Chickpeas (garbanzo), canned, re-heated, drained	100	115	16.1	0	4.1
Navy beans, dried, boiled in unsalted water	100	95	17.2	1	6.1
Lentils, canned in tomato sauce, re-heated	100	55	9.3	1	1.7
Lentils, green and brown, whole, dried, boiled in salted water	100	105	16.9	0	3.8
Lentils, red, split, dried, boiled in unsalted water	100	100	17.5	1	1.9
Red kidney beans, canned, re-heated, drained	100	100	17.8	4	6.2
Soy beans, dried, boiled in unsalted water	100	141	5.1	2	6.1

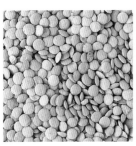
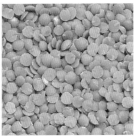
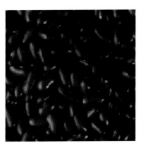
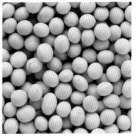

Vegetables

Food	Weight (grams)	Energy (cal)	Carbohydrate (grams)	Sugar (grams)	Fiber (grams)
Alfalfa sprouts, raw	100	24	0.4	0	1.7
Artichoke, Jerusalem, boiled in unsalted water	100	41	10.6	2	3.5
Asparagus, boiled, weighed as served	100	13	0.7	1	0.7
Asparagus, raw	100	25	2	2	1.7
Baked beans, canned in tomato sauce	100	81	15.1	6	3.5
Bamboo shoots, canned, drained	100	11	0.7	1	1.7
Beansprouts, mung, raw	100	31	4	2	1.5
Beets, boiled in salted water	100	46	9.5	9	1.9
Beets, pickled, drained	100	28	5.6	6	1.7
Beets, raw	100	36	7.6	7	1.9
Bell peppers, capsicum, green, raw	100	15	2.6	2	1.6
Bell peppers, capsicum, red, raw	100	32	6.4	6	1.6
Black-eyed peas, dried, raw	100	311	54.1	3	8.2
Breadfruit, canned, drained	100	66	16.4	2	1.7
Fava beans, dried, raw	100	245	32.5	6	27.6
Broccoli, green, boiled in unsalted water	100	24	1.1	1	2.3
Broccoli, green, raw	100	33	1.8	2	2.6
Broccoli, purple sprouting, boiled in unsalted water	100	19	1.3	1	2.3
Broccoli, purple sprouting, raw	100	35	2.6	2	3.5
Brussels sprouts, boiled in unsalted water	100	35	3.5	3	3.1
Lima beans, dried, boiled in unsalted water	100	103	18.4	2	5.2
Cabbage, spring, boiled	100	7	0.8	1	2
Cabbage, winter, boiled	100	15	2.3	2	2.7
Cabbage, Chinese, raw	100	12	1.4	1	1.2
Cabbage, red, raw	100	21	3.7	3	2.5
Cabbage, Savoy, raw	100	27	3.9	4	3.1

Food	Weight (grams)	Energy (cal)	Carbohydrate (grams)	Sugar (grams)	Fiber (grams)
Cabbage, summer, raw	100	24	3.7	4	2
Cabbage, white, raw	100	27	5	5	2.1
Carrot juice	100	24	5.7	6	Trace
Carrots, old, boiled in unsalted water	100	24	4.9	5	2.5
Carrots, young, boiled in unsalted water	100	22	4.4	4	2.3
Carrots, young, raw	100	30	6	6	2.4
Cassava chips	100	353	91.4	6	4
Cassava, baked	100	155	40.1	2	1.7
Cassava, steamed	100	142	36.8	2	1.6
Cauliflower, boiled in unsalted water	100	28	2.1	2	1.6
Cauliflower, frozen, boiled in unsalted water	100	20	2	2	1.2
Celeriac, raw	100	18	2.3	2	3.7
Celery, raw	100	7	0.9	1	1.1
Fries, straight cut, frozen, fried in corn oil	100	273	36	1	2.4
Corn, baby, fresh and frozen, boiled in salted water	100	24	2.7	2	2
Corn, kernels, canned, re-heated, drained	100	122	26.6	10	1.4
Corn, kernels, raw	100	93	17	2	1.5
Corn, on-the-cob, whole, boiled in unsalted water	100	66	11.6	1	1.3
Corn, yellow, cream, canned, regular	100	72	18.1	3.2	1.2
Curly kale, raw	100	33	1.4	1	3.1
Cucumber, raw	100	10	1.5	1	0.6
Eggplant, fried in corn oil	100	302	2.8	3	2.3
Eggplant, raw	100	15	2.2	2	2
Endive, raw	100	13	1	1	2
Escarole	100	11	2.8	1	0.9
Fennel, Florence, raw	100	12	1.8	2	2.4
Garlic, raw	100	98	16.3	2	4.1
Green beans, boiled in unsalted water	100	22	2.9	2	2.4

Food	Weight (grams)	Energy (cal)	Carbohydrate (grams)	Sugar (grams)	Fiber (grams)
Haricot beans, dried, boiled in unsalted water	100	95	17.2	1	6.1
Kohl rabi, raw	100	23	3.7	4	2.2
Leeks, raw	100	22	2.9	2	2.2
Lentils, red, split, dried, raw	100	318	56.3	2	4.9
Lettuce, butterhead, raw	100	12	1.2	1	1.2
Lettuce, Webbs, raw	100	13	2	2	0.8
Lettuce, Romaine, raw	100	16	1.7	2	1.2
Lettuce, Iceberg, raw	100	13	1.9	2	0.6
Marrow, boiled in unsalted water	100	9	1.6	1	0.6
Mixed vegetables, canned, re-heated, drained	100	38	6.1	3	1.7
Mung beans, whole, dried, raw	100	279	46.3	2	10
Mushrooms, common, raw	100	13	0.4	0	1.1
New potatoes, boiled in unsalted water	100	75	17.8	1	1.1
Okra, raw	100	31	3	3	4
Old potatoes, average, raw	100	75	17.2	1	1.3
Onions, raw	100	36	7.9	6	1.4
Parsnip, raw	100	64	12.5	6	4.6
Peas, frozen, raw	100	66	9.3	3	5.1
Peas, raw	100	83	11.3	2	4.7
Pumpkin, raw	100	13	2.2	2	1
Radish, red, raw	100	12	1.9	2	0.9
Red kidney beans, dried, raw	100	266	44.1	3	15.7
Seaweed, nori, dried, raw	100	136	Trace	Trace	44.4
Soy beans, dried, raw100	370	15.8	6	15.7	
Spinach, raw	100	25	1.6	2	2.1
Squash, butternut, baked	100	32	7.4	4	1.4
Squash, spaghetti, baked	100	23	4.3	3	2.1
Sweet potato, baked	100	115	27.9	15	3.3
Tomatoes, canned, whole contents	100	16	3	3	0.7
Tomatoes, cherry, raw	100	18	3	3	1

Food	Weight (grams)	Energy (cal)	Carbohydrate (grams)	Sugar (grams)	Fiber (grams)
Tomatoes, raw	100	17	3.1	3	1
Watercress, raw	100	22	0.4	0	1.5
Yam, baked	100	153	37.5	1	1.7
Zucchini, raw	100	18	1.8	2	0.9
Zucchini, fried in oil	100	63	2.6	3	1.2

Fruit

Food	Weight (grams)	Energy (cal)	Carbohydrate (grams)	Sugar (grams)	Fiber (grams)
Apples, cooking, baked without sugar, flesh and skin	100	45	11.2	11	2
Apples, eating, average, raw	100	47	11.8	12	1.8
Apples, eating, Golden Delicious, raw	100	43	10.8	11	1.7
Apples, eating, Golden Delicious, raw, weighed with core	100	40	9.9	10	1.6
Apples, eating, Granny Smith, raw	100	45	11.5	12	1.7
Apples, eating, red dessert, raw	100	51	13	13	1.9
Apricots, dried	100	188	43.4	43	7.7
Apricots, raw	100	31	7.2	7	1.7
Avocado, average	100	190	1.9	1	3.4
Bananas	100	95	23.2	21	1.1
Blackberries, raw	100	25	5.1	5	3.1
Blackcurrants, raw	100	28	6.6	7	3.6
Breadfruit, canned, drained	100	66	16.4	2	1.7
Carambola	100	32	7.3	7	1.3
Cherries, raw	100	48	11.5	12	0.9
Clementines	100	37	8.7	9	1.2
Cranberries	100	15	3.4	3	3
Damsons, raw	100	38	9.6	10	1.8
Dates, dried	100	270	68	68	4
Dates, raw	100	124	31.3	31	1.8
Dried mixed fruit	100	268	68.1	68	2.2

Food	Weight (grams)	Energy (cal)	Carbohydrate (grams)	Sugar (grams)	Fiber (grams)
Figs, dried	100	227	52.9	53	7.5
Figs, raw	100	43	9.5	10	1.5
Fruit cocktail, canned in juice	100	29	7.2	7	1
Fruit salad, homemade	100	60	14.8	14	1.3
Golden raisins	100	275	69.4	69	2
Gooseberries, cooking, raw	100	19	3	3	2.4
Gooseberries, cooking, stewed without sugar	100	16	2.5	3	2
Gooseberries, dessert, raw	100	40	9.2	9	2.4
Grape juice, unsweetened	100	46	11.7	12	0
Grapefruit juice, unsweetened	100	33	8.3	8	Trace
Grapefruit, raw	100	30	6.8	7	1.3
Grapes, average	100	60	15.4	15	0.7
Greengages, stewed without sugar	100	36	8.7	9	1.9
Grenadillas	100	42	7.5	8	3.3
Guava, raw	100	26	5	5	3.7
Kiwi fruit	100	49	10.6	10	1.9
Kumquats, raw	100	43	9.3	9	3.8
Lemon juice, fresh	100	7	1.6	2	0.1
Lime juice, fresh	100	9	1.6	2	0.1
Loganberries, raw	100	17	3.4	3	2.5
Lychees, raw	100	58	14.3	14	0.7
Mango juice, canned	100	39	9.8	10	Trace
Mandarin oranges, canned in juice	100	32	7.7	8	0.3
Melon, average	100	24	5.5	6	0.7
Melon, Canteloupe-type	100	19	4.2	4	1
Melon, Galia	100	24	5.6	6	0.4
Melon, Honeydew	100	28	6.6	7	0.6
Melon, musk/cantaloupe, raw	100	24	5.3	5	0.6
Melon, watermelon	100	31	7.1	7	0.1
Nectarines	100	40	9	9	1.2
Olives, in brine	100	103	Trace	Trace	2.9
Orange juice, freshly squeezed	100	33	8.1	8	0.1
Orange juice, unsweetened	100	36	8.8	9	0.1

Food	Weight (grams)	Energy (cal)	Carbohydrate (grams)	Sugar (grams)	Fiber (grams)
Oranges	100	37	8.5	9	1.7
Passion fruit	100	36	5.8	6	3.3
Passion fruit juice	100	47	10.7	11	Trace
Paw-paw, raw	100	36	8.8	9	2.2
Peaches, canned in juice	100	39	9.7	10	0.8
Peaches, raw	100	33	7.6	8	1.5
Pears, Comice, raw	100	33	8.5	9	2
Pears, Conference, raw	100	53	13.2	13	2.4
Pears, Nashi, raw	100	29	7.1	7	1.5
Pears, Bartlett, raw	100	34	8.3	8	2.2
Pineapple juice, unsweetened	100	41	10.5	11	Trace
Pineapple, canned in juice	100	47	12.2	12	0.5
Pineapple, raw	100	41	10.1	10	1.2
Plums, Victoria, raw	100	39	9.6	10	1.8
Plums, yellow, raw	100	25	5.9	6	1
Pomegranate	100	51	11.8	12	3.4
Pomegranate juice, fresh	100	44	11.6	12	Trace
Prune juice	100	57	14.4	14	Trace
Prunes	100	160	38.4	38	6.5
Prunes, ready-to-eat	100	141	34	34	5.7
Prunes, stewed without sugar	100	81	19.5	20	3.3
Raisins	100	272	69.3	69	2
Raspberries, frozen	100	26	4.9	5	2.7
Raspberries, raw	100	25	4.6	5	2.5
Redcurrants, raw	100	21	4.4	4	3.4
Rhubarb, stewed without sugar	100	7	0.7	1	1.3
Satsumas	100	36	8.5	9	1.3
Sharon fruit	100	73	18.6	19	1.6
Strawberries, frozen	100	33	7.8	8	1.2
Strawberries, raw	100	27	6	6	1.1
Sultanas	100	275	69.4	69	2
Tangerines	100	35	8	8	1.3
Whitecurrants, raw	100	26	5.6	6	3.4

Dairy

Food	Weight (grams)	Energy (cal)	Carbohydrate (grams)	Sugar (grams)	Fiber (grams)
Coconut milk	100	22	4.9	5	Trace
Condensed milk, skimmed, sweetened	100	267	60	60	0
Condensed milk, whole, sweetened	100	333	55.5	56	0
Dried skim milk, with vegetable fat	100	487	42.6	43	0
Dried whole milk	100	490	39.4	39	0
Evaporated milk, whole	100	151	8.5	9	0
Flavored milk	100	68	10.6	9	0
Goats milk, pasteurized	100	62	4.4	4	0
Low-fat milk, average	100	46	4.7	5	0
Skim milk, average	100	32	4.4	4	0
Soy, non-dairy alternative to milk, unsweetened	100	26	0.5	0	0.2
Soy, non-dairy alternative to milk, sweetened, calcium enriched	100	43	2.5	2	Trace
Whole milk, average	100	66	4.5	5	0
Greek yogurt, cows	100	115	2	2	0
Greek yogurt, sheep	100	92	5	5	0
Low fat yogurt, flavored	100	90	17.9	18	0
Low fat yogurt, muesli/nut	100	112	19.2	18	0
Soy, alternative to yogurt, fruit	100	73	12.9	12	0.3
Whole milk yogurt, fruit	100	109	17.7	17	0
Whole milk yogurt, unflavored	100	79	7.8	8	0
Yogurt, greek style, fruit	100	137	11.2	11	Trace
Yogurt, low fat, unflavored	100	56	7.4	7	0
Yogurt, low fat, fruit	100	78	13.7	13	0.2
Yogurt, virtually fat free fruit	100	47	7	6	Trace
Yogurt, virtually fat free unflavored	100	54	8.2	8	0

Ice Cream

Food	Weight (grams)	Energy (cal)	Carbohydrate (grams)	Sugar (grams)	Fiber (grams)
Baked Alaska	100	200	33.3	25	Trace
Banana split	100	182	19.3	16	0.6
Chocolate covered ice cream bar	100	320	24	23	Trace
Chocolate nut sundae	100	243	26.2	25	0.2
Ice cream, dairy, vanilla	100	177	19.8	19	Trace
Ice cream, vanilla, light	100	165	25.8	22.1	Trace
Ice cream, with cone	100	186	25.5	18	Trace
Kulfi	100	424	11.8	12	0.6

Snacks

Food	Weight (grams)	Energy (cal)	Carbohydrate (grams)	Sugar (grams)	Fiber (grams)
Banana chips	100	519	58.4	35	7.7
Breadsticks	100	392	72.5	5	2.8
Chex Mix	100	425	65.1	not measured	5.6
Corn snacks	100	519	54.3	5	1
Crispy Rice Snacks, peanut butter	100	443	71	32	2.1
Popcorn, candied	100	480	77.6	62	1
Pork rinds	100	606	0.2	0	0.3
Potato and corn sticks	100	462	60.4	2	3.1
Potato chips	100	530	53.3	1	5.3
Potato chips, reduced fat	100	487	67.8	0.2	6.1
Potato chips, jacket	100	510	51.3	1	4.8
Potato chips, low fat	100	458	63.5	2	5.9
Potato chips, thick-cut	100	499	58.0	2	5
Pretzels	100	381	79.2	2	2
Tortilla chips	100	459	60.1	1	6
Trail Mix	100	432	37.2	37	4.3

Candy

Food	Weight (grams)	Energy (cal)	Carbohydrate (grams)	Sugar (grams)	Fiber (grams)
Butterscotch	100	395	95.3	not measured	0
Caramels	100	382	77	66	1.2
Gumdrops, jelly pieces	100	386	98.9	not measured	0
Hard candy	100	394	98	63	0
Hershey, Krackel Choc. Bar	100	531	61.6	51	2.2
Reese's Peanut Butter Cups	100	541	54.6	47	3.2
Reese's Pieces Candy	100	491	61.4	53	2.9
Jellybeans	100	367	93.1	not measured	0
Mini Milk Choc. Candies	100	498	67.1	not measured	2.7
Marshmallows	100	318	81.3	56	0.1
Milk chocolate	100	513	59.2	not measured	3.4
Milk choc. coated raisins	100	390	68.3	62	4.2
Nestlé, Baby Ruth Bar	100	481	65.2	52	2.9
Nestlé, Chunky Bar	100	495	57.1	not measured	4.8
Peanut Chocolate Candies	100	516	60.5	51	3.4
Skittles Original Bite Size Candies	100	405	90.6	76	0
Snickers Bar	100	479	59.2	49	2.5
Starburst Fruit Chews	100	396	84.5	67	0

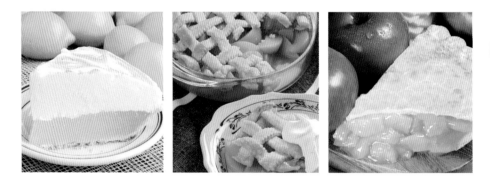

Pies and pastries

Food	Weight (grams)	Energy (cal)	Carbohydrate (grams)	Sugar (grams)	Fiber (grams)
Apple pie, pastry top and bottom	100	266	35.8	14	1.7
Apple pie, wholemeal, pastry top and bottom	100	257	31.9	14	3.4
Fruit pie filling	100	77	20.1	15	1
Fruit pie, pastry top and bottom	100	262	33.9	12	1.7
Fruit pie, wholemeal, pastry top and bottom	100	253	30	12	3.4
Beef Pot Pie, frozen entrée	100	227	22.3	not measured	1.1
Stouffer's Chicken Pie, frozen entrée	100	202	12.9	not measured	1.1
Pie, vegetable, wholemeal	100	146	16.5	3	2.5
Pie, vegetable	100	159	18.8	3	1.5
Pierre, Flame Broiled Meatloaf	100	219	5.3	2	0.7
Turkey Pot Pie, frozen entrée	100	176	17.7	not measured	1.1

Desserts

Food	Weight (grams)	Energy (cal)	Carbohydrate (grams)	Sugar (grams)	Fiber (grams)
Cheesecake	100	426	24.6	14	0.4
Creme caramel	100	104	20.6	18	0
Custard, egg	100	118	11	11	0
Custard, made up with low fat milk	100	94	16.8	12	Trace
Frozen ice cream desserts	100	251	21	20	Trace
Fruit fool	100	163	20.2	16	1.2
Jello, made with water	100	61	15.1	15	0
Mousse, chocolate	100	149	19.9	18	Trace
Mousse, fruit	100	143	18	18	0.4
Trifle	100	166	21	17	0.4
Pavlova, with fruit and cream	100	288	42.2	41	0.3
Profiteroles with sauce	100	346	24.6	17	Trace

Drinks

Food	Weight (grams)	Energy (cal)	Carbohydrate (grams)	Sugar (grams)	Fiber (grams)
Cola, contains caffeine	100	41	10.75	10.75	0
Cola, without caffeine	100	41	10.75	10.75	0
Root beer	100	41	10.6	11	0
Cream soda	100	51	13.3	not measured	0
Lemon-lime soda	100	40	10.4	not measured	0
Lemon-lime, with caffeine	100	41	10.4	not measured	0
Soda, club	100	0	0	not measured	0
Fruit juice drink, ready to drink	100	37	9.8	10	Trace
Fruit drink, low calorie, concentrated, made up	100	1	0.2	0	0
Fruit drink, concentrated, made up	100	19	5	5	0
Fruit drink, concentrated, made up	100	19	5	5	0
Low calorie, cola, with aspartame, contains caffeine	100	1	0.1	not measured	0
Low calorie, cola or pepper-types, with sodium saccharin, contains caffeine	100	0	0.1	not measured	0

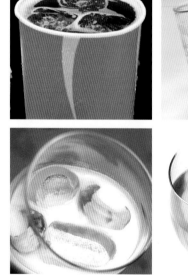
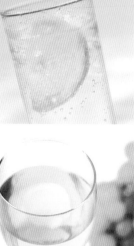
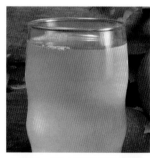
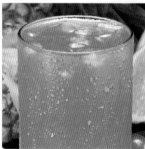

Alcohol

Food	Weight (grams)	Energy (cal)	Carbohydrate (grams)	Sugar (grams)	Fiber (grams)
Beer, light	100	28	1.3	not measured	0
Beer, regular	100	41	3.7	not measured	0.2
Champagne	100	76	1.4	1	0
Cherry brandy	100	255	32.6	33	0
Cider, low alcohol	100	17	3.6	4	0
Cider, sweet	100	42	4.3	4	0
Cream liqueurs	100	325	22.8	23	0
Creme de Menthe, 72 proof	100	371	41.6	41.6	0
Curacao	100	311	28.3	28	0
Daiquiri, canned	100	125	15.7	not measured	0
Egg nog	100	114	9.8	10	0
gin, rum, vodka, whiskey 100 proof	100	295	0	not measured	0
gin, rum, vodka, whiskey 94 proof	100	275	0	not measured	0
gin, rum, vodka, whiskey 90 proof	100	263	0	not measured	0
gin, rum, vodka, whiskey 86 proof	100	250	0	not measured	0
gin, rum, vodka, whiskey 80 proof	100	231	0	not measured	0
Lager, bottled	100	29	1.5	2	0
Liqueur, coffee with cream, 63 proof	100	308	32.2	not measured	0
Liqueur, coffee with cream, 53 proof	100	336	46.8	not measured	0
Liqueur, coffee with cream, 34 proof	100	327	20.9	not measured	0
Liqueurs, high strength	100	314	24.4	24	0
Liqueurs, low-medium strength	100	262	32.8	33	0
Martini, prepared from recipe	100	243	2.04	0.19	0
Port	100	157	12	12	0
Red wine	100	72	1.7	0	0
Rose wine, medium	100	71	2.5	3	0
Sake	100	134	5.0	0	0
Sherry, dry	100	116	1.4	1	0
Sherry, sweet	100	136	6.9	7	0
White wine, dry	100	66	0.6	1	0
White wine, medium	100	74	3	3	0
White wine, sparkling	100	74	5.1	5	0
White wine, sweet	100	94	5.9	6	0
Wine, light	100	50	1.17	1.15	0
Vanilla extract, imitation, alcohol	100	237	2.4	not measured	0

Index

Further reading

Jane Kirby. Dieting for Dummies. John Wiley & Sons Inc., 2004

Anita Bean. Food for Fitness: Nutrition Plan, Eating Plan Recipes. A & C Black, 2002.

Robert C. Atkins. Atkins for Life: the Controlled Diet for Permanent Weight Loss and Good Health. Pan, 2003.

> Website: www.atkins.com

Barry Spears. The 7-day Zone Diet: Join the Low Carb Revolution. Harper Collins, 2203

> Website: www.zone.com

Arthur Agatson. The South Beach Diet: A Doctor's Plan for Fast and Lasting Weight Loss. Headline, 2003

Rachael Heller and Richard Heller. The Carbohydrate Addicts Diet. Vermillion, 2000

Helen Foster. Easy GI Diet. Hamlyn, 2004

Azmina Govindji and Nina Puddefoot. The Gi Points Diet. Vermillion, 2004

Wynnie Chan. Food and Diet Counter: Complete Nutritional Facts for Every Diet. Hamlyn, 2003.

American Dietetic Association and Roberta Larson Duyff (editor). 365 days of Healthy Eating. John Wiley & Sons Ltd

Leighton H. Steward, Morrison C. Bethea, Sam S. Andrews, and Luis A. Balart. Sugar Busters! Cut Sugar to Trim Fat. I B S Books, 1998

Rick Gallop. The G.I. Diet: The Easy Healthy Way to Permanent Weight Loss. Workman publishing, 2003

Anita Bean. The Complete Guide to Sports Nutrition. 4th edition. A & C Black, 2003

Nutrient data has been obtained from McCance and Widdowson's The Composition of Foods, 6th Edition, The Royal Society of Chemistry, and the Food Standards Agency, 2003

Acknowledgments

All images © Chrysalis Image Library apart from the following.

B = Bottom C= Center T= Top L = Left R = Right

© **Digital Vision** 17BL, 18L, 20L, 62L, 63TL, 64BR, 93L, 94TC, 127R.

© **Digital Stock** 29R, 33BL,34TR, 34BL, 34BR, 46, 47BR, 54R, 55L, 55R, 56TR, 56BL, 58L, 63CR, 64TR, 65L, 65R, 73L, 73R, 74, 74C, 75C, 76L, 76C, 142L, 143CL, 154, 156TL, 156TC, 156TR, 156BL, 156BC.

© **Stockbyte** 1, 2, 7, 8L, 10BL, 10BR, 11, 12R, 14TL, 14BL, 15C, 15R, 17TL, 22C, 23TC, 23TR, 23BL, 24C, 24R, 25, 26TL, 26CR, 26BR, 29L, 29CL, 29CR, 30TL, 30T, 30BL, 30BR, 31TL, 31C, 31TR, 31BR, 32L, 32C, 32R, 33TL, 33TC, 33BC, 33BR, 34TL, 34CL, 34CR, 35L, 35C, 35R, 37, 38L, 38R, 40R, 43TL, 43BR, 44TL, 45, 46C, 46R, 47TL, 48TL, 48TR, 48BL, 48BR, 49L, 50L, 50R, 51L, 51R, 53, 54L, 56TL, 56BR, 57, 58C, 58R, 59L, 59C, 59R, 61BC, 61BR, 62C, 62R, 63TR, 63CL, 63BL, 64TL, 64BL, 66, 68L, 68TR, 68CR, 68BR, 69TC, 69TR, 69BC, 69BR, 70T, 71, 72TL, 72BL, 73C, 74R, 75L, 75R, 76R, 77, 85TL, 85BL, 86L, 87R, 89C, 90L, 91BC, 92CL, 92BR, 94TL, 94TR, 94BL, 94BC, 95L, 95R, 100BL, 101, 113R, 114L, 114, 114R, 116L, 116C, 118L, 118C, 119L, 119R, 120L, 120C, 120R, 122, 123L, 123C, 123R, 127C, 131L, 131R, 132L, 132R, 134C, 140L, 140C, 141.

Chrysalis Books Group Plc is committed to respecting the intellectual property rights of others. We have therefore taken all reasonable efforts to ensure that the reproduction of all content on these pages is done with the full consent of copyright owners. If you are aware of any unintentional omissions please contact the company directly so that any necessary corrections may be made for future editions.